Pocket Essential Medical Equipment

Pocket Series

About the Series

This series of highly-practical and portable pocket books provide concise and reader-friendly guidance for medical students and junior doctors across a variety of subjects for use in a range of clinical settings.

Pocket On Call, 1E
Andrew Stewart

Pocket Clinical Examiner, 1E
Adam Barnett, Thomas Bannister

Pocket Essential Medical Equipment, 1E
Norbert Banhidy, David Zhang

For more information about this series please visit: https://www.routledge.com/Pocket-Series/book-series/CRCPOCKETSER

Pocket Essential Medical Equipment

Norbert Banhidy
and David Zhang

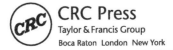

CRC Press
Taylor & Francis Group
Boca Raton London New York

CRC Press is an imprint of the
Taylor & Francis Group, an **informa** business

First edition published 2022

by CRC Press
6000 Broken Sound Parkway NW, Suite 300, Boca Raton, FL 33487-2742

and by CRC Press
2 Park Square, Milton Park, Abingdon, Oxon, OX14 4RN

Library of Congress Cataloging-in-Publication Data
A catalog record for this title has been requested

ISBN: 9780367747145 (hbk)
ISBN: 9780367745783 (pbk)
ISBN: 9781003159179 (ebk)

DOI: 10.1201/9781003159179

Typeset in Goudy Oldstyle Std
by KnowledgeWorks Global Ltd.

To my grandfather

NB

To Louise, Evan and my parents,
Qinghua and Tusheng Zhang

DZ

Contents

Preface

Modern medicine would not be where it is today, were it not for the innovations in medical technology and the abundance of medical equipment available to healthcare professionals. Depending on the specialty, the average healthcare professional will use multiple types of medical equipment to aid in the diagnosis or treatment of disease, or the monitoring of patients' health. Adequate knowledge of the equipment, and its safe use, is therefore essential to delivering effective and safe patient care. It is somewhat surprising, therefore, that often healthcare professionals are unfamiliar with the use (or even unaware of the existence) of the medical or surgical equipment they may need to use, right up until the point they are required to perform the procedure.

To address this issue, this book aims to serve as an illustrative guide for commonly used medical and surgical equipment found on the wards, clinics and in A&E. We hope this book will serve as a reference tool for medical students and junior doctors alike, who may not have come across the equipment before or are not familiar with their exact indications and correct use. Using this book will allow students and doctors to familiarise themselves with the equipment before having to use them in a clinical setting, thereby hopefully increasing readers' knowledge and confidence in subsequent clinical situations.

Given the almost inexhaustible list of medical equipment in existence, certain items have had to be prioritised and thus only a list of the most used every-day equipment are presented in this book. The book does not contain specific surgical instruments used in the operating theatre, nor does it aim to describe the use of large and often complex medical devices such as ventilators or X-ray machines.

We hope this book will serve you well in preparation for your exams or clinical rotations, and ultimately enrich the experience of your journey through clinical practice.

NB and DZ

Acknowledgements

We would like to thank our senior publisher, Dr Joanna Koster of CRC Press, for her invaluable role in guiding us through the whole process from the book's conception to its publication.

We would also like to thank all the clinical teams at the Royal London Hospital, Barts Health NHS Trust for providing the equipment for the photographs.

We are grateful to London's Air Ambulance Charity, especially Mr Bill Leaning, for allowing us to take photos of their trauma management equipment.

How to use this book

This book is intended both for those who wish to systematically learn about all of the equipment across different specialties and those who simply want to use it as a handy reference guide when on the wards.

The equipment is organised into chapters based on specialty and body system.

Each medical equipment section is set in the following way:

1. A brief **description** detailing the equipment's general purpose and its components
2. A list of **indications** outlining the equipment's most common uses
3. A brief description of the equipment's **directions of use**
4. A summary of **cautions and contraindications** to be aware and ensure safe use
5. Finally, an accompanying photograph of the equipment to facilitate learning

List of abbreviations

A&E	Accident and Emergency
ABCDE	Airway, Breathing, Circulation, Disability, Exposure
ABG	Arterial Blood Gas
ALS	Advanced Life Support
ATLS	Adult Trauma Life Support
AV	Arterio-venous
BiPAP	Bilevel Positive Airway Pressure
BTS	British Thoracic Society
C	Cervical
CAT	Combat Application Tourniquet
CO_2	Carbon Dioxide
COPD	Chronic Obstructive Pulmonary Disorder
COVID	Coronavirus Disease
CPAP	Continuous Positive Airway Pressure
CSF	Cerebrospinal Fluid
CT	Computed Tomography
CVC	Central Venous Catheter
DNAR	Do Not Attempt to Resuscitate
DVT	Deep Venous Thrombosis
ECG	Electrocardiogram
ENT	Ear, Nose and Throat
ETI	Endotracheal Tube Introducer
ETT	Endotracheal Tube
FAST	Focussed Assessment with Sonography for Trauma
FiO_2	Fraction of Inspired Oxygen
Fr	French (medical tubing unit of measurement)

GCS	Glasgow Coma Scale
GI	Gastrointestinal
HAS	Human Albumin Solution
Hz	Hertz
ICP	Intracranial Pressure
IO	Intraosseous
ITU	Intensive Treatment Unit
IV	Intravenous
L	Lumbar
LMA	Laryngeal Mask Airway
NG	Nasogastric
NIV	Non-invasive Ventilation
NPA	Nasopharyngeal Airway
OHS	Obesity Hypoventilation Syndrome
OPA	Oropharyngeal Airway
OSA	Obstructive Sleep Apnoea
PaCO$_2$	Partial Pressure of Carbon Dioxide
PaO$_2$	Partial Pressure of Oxygen
POP	Plaster of Paris
PPE	Personal Protective Equipment
S	Sacral
STI	Sexually Transmitted Infection
TUR	Transurethral Resection
UTI	Urinary Tract Infection
VBG	Venous Blood Gas
VF	Ventricular Fibrillation
VT	Ventricular Tachycardia
VTE	Venous Thromboembolism

About the authors

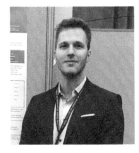

Norbert Banhidy is a core surgical trainee in London, UK

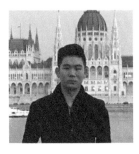

David Zhang is an internal medicine trainee in London, UK

Section I

Resuscitation "ABCDE" equipment

Airway

Nasopharyngeal airway

Description:

- A flexible rubber tube consisting of a smooth angled tip, curved body and flanged end which can be inserted into the nose and extends into the top of the oropharynx
- Sizes range from 2 to 9 (corresponding to diameter in mm) with male adults usually requiring size 7 to 8 and females 6 to 7

Indication:

- Airway adjunct used to provide an airway in patients with an intact gag reflex, trismus or oral trauma
- May be used instead of or in conjunction with an oropharyngeal airway (see *Oropharyngeal airway*)

Directions of use:

- Select appropriate nostril for insertion (typically right nostril) and apply local anaesthetic spray
- Apply lubricant to tube and insert with bevel facing the nasal septum

DOI: 10.1201/9781003159179-2

- Advance along the septum horizontally, following the natural curvature of the floor of the nasopharyngeal cavity and rotated 90 degrees to lie in the nasopharynx
- Safety pin may be placed behind flange to prevent the advancement of tube
- Correct position can be confirmed by visualising tube tip behind uvula

Cautions and contraindications:

- Major contraindication is base of skull fractures due to possible intracranial placement
- Main complications include epistaxis, ulceration, infection, blockage

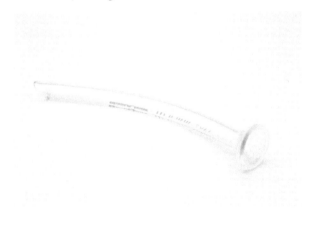

Oropharyngeal airway

Description:

- Also known as "Guedel" airway
- Rigid plastic tube inserted into mouth, curved to sit along the roof of the oral cavity and end at the tongue base
- Sizes are colour coded for easy identification (children – 0, 1, 2; adults – 4, 5, 6)

Indication:

- Airway adjunct used to lift the tongue off the posterior pharyngeal wall to prevent airway obstruction in reduced GCS (≤8)
- Also allows for oropharyngeal suctioning

Directions of use:

- Identify the correct size by measuring from the centre of the mouth between the first incisors to the angle of the mandible in an adult
- Ensure no foreign bodies in the oral cavity
- Lubricate the oropharyngeal airway
- Insert into the mouth upside down (reduces risk of pushing tongue back)
- Once tip is around the hard-soft palate junction, rotate 180 degrees and advance until flange at mouth opening
- Confirm airway patency

Cautions and contraindications:

- The main contraindication is use in patients with intact gag reflex (GCS>8)
- Main complications include gagging, vomiting and aspiration; soft tissue trauma to the tongue, palate and pharynx and injury to the teeth

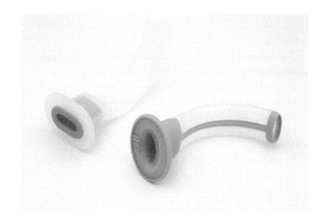

Laryngeal mask airway

Description:
- Supraglottic airway device consisting of flexible plastic tube with an inflatable circular cuff on end which sits above the larynx
- Sizes range from 0 (infant) to 6 (large adult), with typically size 3 or 4 being used for female and male adults, respectively

Indication:
- Ventilation during elective anaesthesia with low risk of aspiration
- Cardiac arrest pre-intubation
- Failed endotracheal tube insertion/lack of available trained staff

Directions of use:
- Select correct size LMA
- Deflate cuff using 20ml syringe
- Lubricate cuff
- Position patient with 15 degree neck flexion and full head extension
- Insert the LMA over the tongue until it reaches the posterior pharynx wall
- Inflate the cuff with 20–40ml of air

Cautions and contraindications:
- Relative contraindications include poor mouth opening; potential pharyngeal/laryngeal pathology and high airway resistance
- Main complications include inability to achieve a seal and sufficient ventilation; aspiration; malposition and dislodgement

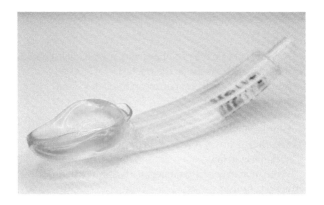

Endotracheal tube

Description:
- A flexible plastic tube equipped with an inflatable cuff on the end which sits inside the trachea
- Size typically used: 8mm diameter for males, 7mm diameter for females

Indication:
- Ventilation during anaesthesia for major surgery
- Securing of airway (GCS<8, airway burns, epiglottitis, neck haematoma)
- Ventilation in severe respiratory pathology (COPD, ARDS)

Directions of use:
- Note that ET tube placement should only be attempted by appropriately trained healthcare professionals
- Select appropriate size ETT
- Lubricate tube
- Direct visualisation of glottis using laryngoscope (see *Laryngoscope*)
- Insert ETT through the vocal cords to sit in the trachea
- Inflate ETT cuff

Cautions and contraindications:
- Relative contraindications include severe airway trauma or obstruction preventing ETT placement, severe cervical spine injury which requires complete immobilisation
- Main complications include trauma to teeth/gums, bleeding, cuff perforation, malposition and dislodgement. Late complications include infection and tracheal stenosis.

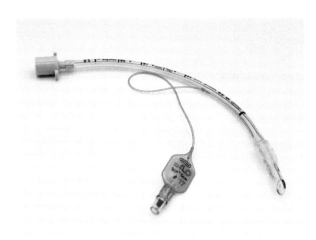

Suction kit

Description:
- Device used to create negative pressure to achieve suctioning of airway, consisting of vacuum source, collection canister, tubing and suction tip
- Suction device may be wall-mounted by patient's bedside or portable
- Various suction tips are available that may be attached to suction device including the Yankauer suction tip or the non-rigid whistle tip suction catheter

Indication:
- Removal of airway contents including blood, saliva, vomit or other secretions
- May also be used in surgery to remove blood or other fluids from the operative field of view

Directions of use:
- Attach appropriate suction tip to tube connected to suction device
- Select appropriate suction pressure (100–150mmHg for adults and 80–100mmHg for infants) and check suction by momentarily occluding suction tip with finger
- Apply suction tip to visible areas only

Cautions and contraindications:
- Complications include mucosal damage, device blockage or equipment failure

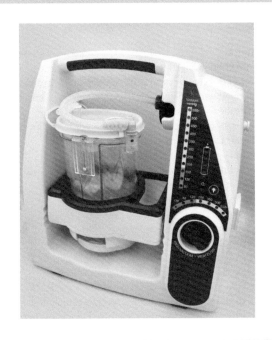

Tracheostomy tube

Description:
- Curved hollow plastic tube with flanged opening which is inserted through front of neck access and sits in trachea
- Key components include a rigid outer tube and a removable inner tube to aid cleaning and relief of obstruction
- Tracheostomy tube sizes vary between different types and different manufacturers

Indication:
- Front of neck airway access in "cannot intubate, cannot oxygenate" (CICO) situations
- Post-intubation ventilation weaning
- Post-laryngectomy
- Patients at high risk of pulmonary aspiration

Directions of use:
- The surgical procedure of emergency and elective tracheostomy fall outside the scope of this book
- Insertion and changing of tracheostomies should be managed sufficiently by trained specialists including ENT surgeons, anaesthetists and speech and language therapists

Cautions and contraindications:
- Complications may be categorised into immediate, delayed and late:
  - Immediate complications include damage to local structures, malposition, surgical emphysema or pneumothorax
  - Delayed complications include infection, tube migration, mucosal ulceration, obstruction
  - Late complications include tracheal stenosis, fistulation, psychological effects

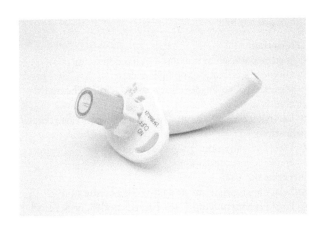

Laryngoscope

Description:
- Instrument used to visualise larynx, consisting of a curved blade, handle and light source
- Various types of blades exist – the Macintosh being the commonest
- Laryngoscopes may be attached to a fibreoptic video output

Indication:
- Direct visualisation of the vocal cords to aid endotracheal intubation

Directions of use:
- Select appropriate size and blade for examination
- Position patient lying down, head extended, neck flexed
- Position yourself at the patient's head
- Non-dominant hand holding handle of laryngoscope
- Carefully slide blade over patient's tongue so that tip of blade sits in the vallecula
- Lift the blade infero-anteriorly until vocal cords are visualised

Cautions and contraindications:
- Absolute contraindications include grade III trismus (inter-incisoral distance of <1cm) and in cases of laryngeal trauma where direct laryngoscopy may further worsen the already existing injury
- Complications include damage to local structures such as teeth, lips, oropharynx, larynx and trachea as well as damage to vocal cords
- Laryngoscopy may also precipitate a sympathetic surge causing tachycardia, arrhythmia, hypertension and in rare cases myocardial ischaemia/infarction

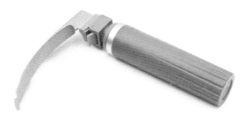

Endotracheal tube introducer (ETI)

Description:

- Flexible plastic stylet ranging between 50 and 60cm in length with distal curved tip which allows passage through the vocal cords during intubation
- Various types exist, most common of which is the Eschmann tracheal tube introducer, also referred to as a "bougie"

Indication:

- Aid in difficult intubation where vocal cords may not be directly visible
- Endotracheal tube exchange
- Adjunct for surgical cricothyroidotomy

Directions of use:

- During intubation, laryngoscopy blade inserted into mouth to aid visualisation of vocal cords (see *Laryngoscope*)
- ETI advanced along blade with curved tip pointing anteriorly under the epiglottis, sliding into the trachea
- Confirmation of correct placement of ETI may be indicated by tactile "clicks" as tip of ETI slides over tracheal rings, or by inability to pass ETI further as airways become smaller
- Endotracheal tube may then be passed over ETI using Seldinger technique and the ETI removed once ETT in place

Cautions and contraindications:

- Complications may include trauma to the airway, damage to vocal cords/arytenoids, malpositioning in oesophagus and failure of procedure

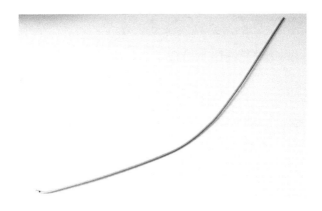

Breathing

Bag valve mask

Description:
- Self-inflating resuscitation device comprising of an elastic bag which re-expands automatically after being manually compressed
- Typically consists of a face mask, self-inflating bag attached to a reservoir bag and an oxygen inlet
- Various sizes are available for infants, children and adults

Indication:
- Provision of controlled manual ventilation
- Assistance of spontaneous ventilation

Directions of use:
- Select appropriate bag size along with correct mask size
- Attach high flow (15L/min) oxygen to the system
- Place mask over mouth and nose and ensure tight seal
- Open airway using two-handed jaw thrust, with assistant delivering well-timed effective compressions to self-inflating bag

DOI: 10.1201/9781003159179-3

Cautions and contraindications:

- Main complications include inadvertent hyperventilation; air leak from poor seal around mask; gastric distension and barotrauma

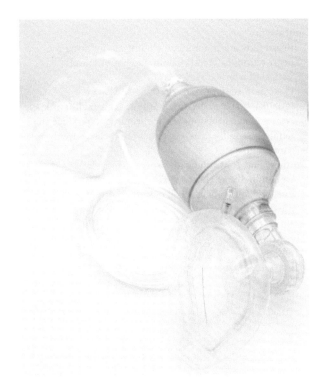

Stethoscope

Description:
- Acoustic device used for the auscultation of internal sounds of the human body
- Typically consists of a disc shaped metal resonator connected to two ear pieces by rubber tubing

Indication:
- Broad indications for use, including auscultating the heart murmurs, breath sounds and bowel sounds

Direction of use:
- Place earpieces into ears
- Push diaphragm or bell firmly against skin and listen closely
- Note some instructions may be required to produce the required sound, e.g. asking patient to breathe deeply through mouth

Cautions and contraindications:
- Generally the stethoscope poses no risk to patients
- Ensure diaphragm and bell of stethoscope cleaned after use on patient

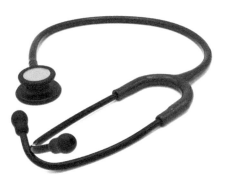

Non-rebreather mask

Description:
- Device consists of mask, designed to overly and form a seal over both nose and mouth, held in place using an elastic cord
- Attached is a reservoir bag, connected to an external oxygen supply
- As the patient breathes out, air is exhaled through a one way valve
- As the patient inhales, high concentration oxygen is inhaled from the reservoir bag
- Patients will generally receive around 60–80% oxygen

Indication:
- Non-rebreather masks deliver high flow oxygen, without aiding breathing
- The most common indication is hypoxia, common in conditions such as pneumonia, asthma and pulmonary embolism
- Other indications include cluster headache and carbon monoxide poisoning

Directions of use:
- Attach oxygen supply at 15L/min to non-rebreather mask
- Seal valve to inflate reservoir bag, ensuring two-third inflation
- Form a tight seal with the mask over patient's nose and mouth and fix in place using elastic cord behind patient's head
- Check oxygen saturations following administration

Caution and contraindication:

- Note if the reservoir bag becomes deflated, the patient will no longer have a source of air to breathe
- Patients with chronically raised carbon dioxide levels may experience CO_2 retention secondary to loss of hypoxic drive
- This is common in patients with diseases such as COPD, OHS and OSA
- Please note that masks are often generic and disposable, therefore a tight seal will not be possible for all facial structures, allowing variable amounts of air to leak in
- Patients may experience claustrophobia or injuries surrounding the mouth from prolonged use

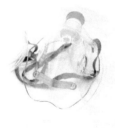

Nebuliser

Description:
- Devices used to aerosolise liquids for inhalation, using compressed air at high velocity
- Commonly used nebulisers are jet nebulisers, ultrasonic wave nebulisers and vibrating mesh nebulisers
- Jet nebulisers achieve aerosolisation using compressed air at high velocity passed through the liquid
- Ultrasonic wave nebulisers generate ultrasonic waves causing vibration and subsequent vaporisation of liquid
- Vibrating mesh technology requires ultrasonic vibration of a fine mesh above liquid to generate the same effect

Indications:
- Delivery of bronchodilatory medications such as salbutamol and ipratropium bromide in cases of pulmonary conditions such as asthma or COPD
- May also be used in the management of airway oedema to deliver nebulised adrenaline
- Management of upper aerodigestive tract secretions by delivering nebulised saline

Directions of use:
- The most common form of nebuliser is the jet nebuliser
- Attach jet nebuliser to liquid reservoir and connect system to a mask, forming a tight seal around the patient's mouth and nose
- Turn on jet nebuliser and begin aerosolisation

Cautions and contraindication:
- Delivery of nebulised medication may cause increased side effects as compared with typical inhaler delivery

- Therefore caution must be used in those with susceptibility to tachyarrhythmias, and those with labile blood pressures
- Note nebulisers may have reduced effect in those with reduced consciousness levels, due to a reduced respiratory drive
- Nebulisation is an aerosol generating procedure and may aid the transmission of respiratory infections

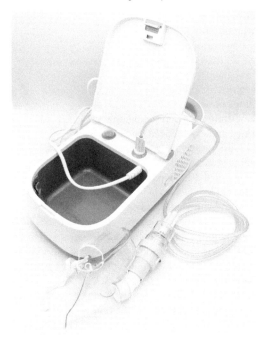

Chest drain

Description:
- Device inserted into the thorax, allowing drainage of fluid or removal of air
- Insertion of chest drain creates a one way system preventing entrance of external air or fluid
- The device itself consists of a hollow chest tube attached to a cylindrical water container

Indication:
- Pneumothorax
- Tension pneumothorax
- Pleural effusion
- Empyema
- Haemopneumothorax

Directions of use:
- Chest drain insertion should only be attempted by trained and experienced medical staff
- Chest drains may be inserted via a surgical approach or Seldinger technique
- The detailed directions of insertion are beyond the scope of this book

Cautions and contraindications:
- Complications include disconnection or accidental removal of chest drain, drain site infection, blockage of chest drain
- Chest drain container should be checked regularly for swinging of the water level to ensure correct position of the drain
- Be aware for re-expansion pulmonary oedema, do not drain more than 1500ml at one time
- Clamping chest drains should be done cautiously

- Pneumothorax should be swinging and bubbling, and should never be clamped whilst bubbling, can lead to tension pneumothorax

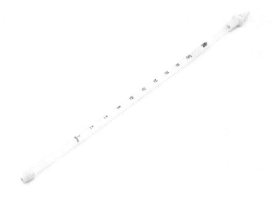

Nasal cannula

Description:
- Device used to deliver oxygen rich air intranasally
- Consists of two plastic nasal prongs, attached to a plastic tube connected to oxygen supply

Indication:
- Hypoxia requiring low levels of supplementary oxygen can be initiated on oxygen therapy via nasal cannulae

Directions of use:
- Attach tubing to an oxygen source
- Set oxygen flow rate to desired level
- Place nasal prongs into nostrils and secure tubing over ears
- Instruct patient to breathe through nose

Cautions and contraindications:
- Patients with facial injuries may not tolerate nasal cannulae
- Patients with blockages of the nasal canals will be unable to receive oxygen therapy using this method
- Note nasal cannulae can only deliver oxygen 4L/min, therefore profound hypoxia should be treated with other methods of oxygen delivery
- Prolonged use of nasal cannulae may lead to local nasal skin breakdown and ulceration

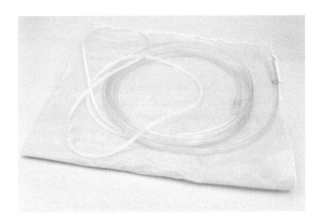

Pulse oximeter

Description:
- Device measuring the saturation of oxygen in circulating haemoglobin
- Pulse oximeter is generally made up of a small plastic clip which can be attached onto the finger
- The clip uses two wavelengths of light passed through a finger to measure peripheral oxygen saturations using a sensor
- The sensor detects pulsating arterial blood and excludes venous blood and other tissues

Indication:
- Pulse oximetry is a fast and effective way to detect hypoxia and measure heart rate
- Furthermore, in medical settings, pulse oximetry is measured as part of routine observation of the patient
- Pulse oximetry provides real time oxygen saturation levels allowing for close monitoring of perfusion and gas exchange

Directions of use:
- Open device and place over the patient's finger
- Allow time for sensor to calibrate and register the oxygen saturation
- Ensure that the finger is warm and well perfused

Cautions and contraindications:
- Certain areas at the peripheries may be poorly perfused and may not reflect central oxygen saturation levels in blood, for such patients the pulse oximeter should be attached elsewhere on the body

- Take caution that pulse oximetry does not give blood CO_2 concentrations, and cannot be used to replace arterial blood sampling in patients with pulmonary diseases
- Heart rate measurement may not be reliable in cases of atrial fibrillation or poor tissue perfusion

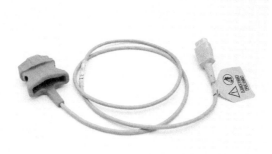

Venturi kit

Description:

- Mask and interchangeable mask valve allowing delivery of high flow oxygen to be delivered at accurate FiO_2 levels depending on the corresponding valve selection
- Valves are colour coded to allow the selection of varying oxygen concentration delivery ranging incrementally from 24 to 60% oxygen

Indications:

- Delivery of controlled levels of oxygen is most commonly indicated in hypoxic patients with chronic hypercapnia (CO_2 retainers), in conditions such as COPD
- Venturi mask allows for accurate measurement of oxygen requirement, not achieved by nasal cannulae

Directions of use:

- Attach mask to specific FiO_2 Venturi attachment
- Using elastic cord, secure mask around patient's head
- Attach oxygen source to Venturi attachment and instruct the patient to breathe as normal
- Please note that differing FiO_2 percentages will require differing rates of oxygen flow as noted on the valves

Cautions and contraindications:

- In cases of COPD, due to loss of hypoxic drive, inappropriately high concentration of oxygen delivered to these patients may lead to cessation of respiration and increase in CO_2 retention and acidosis

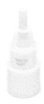
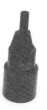
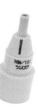

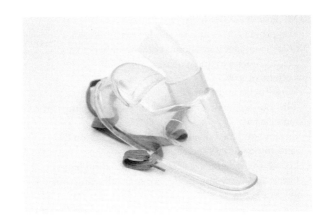

Arterial blood gas kit

Description:
- Small 5ml syringe attached to a 20 gauge, 1.25 inch needle
- Syringe contains small amount of heparin to prevent clot formation of blood sample
- Syringe tip will often be compatible with applicator of blood gas analysis machine

Indication:
- Hypoxic patients will require ABG analysis, to give accurate readings of arterial PaO_2, $PaCO_2$, pH, bicarbonate and base excess
- This is important to distinguish between type 1 and type 2 respiratory failure and can aid stratification of severity of pulmonary diseases
- Modern day ABG (and VBG) analysis will often also provide other information, such as oxygen saturation, lactate, sodium, potassium, haemoglobin, methaemoglobin and glucose

Directions of use:
- Wash hands and wear gloves
- The most common artery used for ABG sampling is the radial artery
- Ensure hand has adequate collateral circulation by performing Allen's test
- Locate the radial pulse using index and third finger
- Clean the area using an alcohol swab, allowing time for alcohol to dry
- Local anaesthetic administration may be advised prior to ABG sampling

- Using the radial pulse as a guide, insert needle into the radial artery
- The syringe should self-fill and pulse with arterial blood
- Remove needle once the syringe is full and apply pressure using gauze and tape
- Replace safety cover onto needle and take sample to gas machine for analysis
- Ensure that the sample does not clot by moving the sample regularly

Cautions and contraindications:

- ABG sampling is uncomfortable and can be painful, BTS guidelines now recommend use of anaesthetic prior to ABG sampling
- Local infection prohibits arterial blood sampling
- Peripheral vascular disease present in limbs may distort results
- One should avoid ABG measurement in arms with AV fistulae
- Severe coagulopathy or thrombolysis are also contraindications to ABG

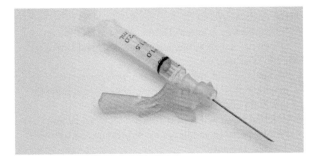

Circulation

DOI: 10.1201/9781003159179-4

Blood pressure cuff

Description:
- Inflatable cuff placed around the arm, allowing readings of blood pressure through blood pressure machine readings or manual methods (using stethoscope)
- Cuffs are available in various paediatric and adult sizes

Indication:
- Blood pressure monitoring forms part of the standard observations required in regular monitoring of patients in the medical setting
- Blood pressure is especially important to monitor in emergencies such as haemorrhage, sepsis and stroke

Directions of use:
- Manual method, inflate the blood pressure cuff to maximal pressure and use stethoscope to auscultate for brachial pulse, slowly deflating
- Brachial pulse will appear at pressures equal to the systolic pressure and disappear at pressures equal to the diastolic pressure

- Blood pressure should be repeated 3 times in order to prevent inaccurate measurements
- Digital blood pressure machines allow automated process of reading blood pressure

Cautions and contraindications:

- There are very few contraindications to measurement of blood pressure
- Inaccurate measurements may be obtained in cases of peripheral lymphoedema
- Arteriovenous fistulae should be avoided, and the other arm should be used
- Fractures or breaches in skin should also be avoided
- Please note that blood pressure measurement may be inaccurately low or high if the cuff used is too small or large respectively

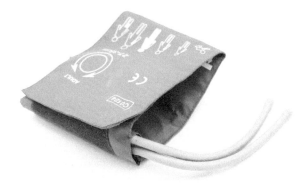

Arterial line

Description:

- Hollow catheter inserted into the artery using Seldinger technique, allowing real time blood pressure monitoring and arterial blood sampling
- Arterial line packs typically include appropriate-sized arterial catheter, corresponding introducer needle, guidewire, lidocaine, gauze tissue, sterile gloves, mask and gowns and chlorhexidine solution for aseptic cleansing
- Line is typically inserted into the radial artery but can in theory be inserted into any artery with collateral circulation

Indication:

- Monitor blood pressure in real time, rather than regular intermittent time intervals, and easily obtain arterial blood sampling
- Typically used in the emergency, anaesthetic or intensive care setting

Directions of use:

- Wash hands carefully and prepare equipment
- Locate radial artery by palpation and perform the Allen's test to ascertain collateral circulation
- Puncture radial artery with introducer needle
- Once pulsatile blood flow is detected, insert the guidewire through the introducer needle
- Once the guidewire is sufficiently advanced, removed the introducer needle

- Thread the arterial catheter over the guidewire, sliding it until it is completely flush with the skin
- Remove the guidewire, inspecting for complete integrity of the tip
- Attach the arterial line set to transducer and monitor in order to observe blood pressure and arterial trace waveform

Cautions and contraindications:

- Absolute contraindications include peripheral vascular disease causing reduced perfusion; local infection to skin; poor collateral blood flow or recent cannulation of collateral artery in limb
- Arterial line insertion is not advised in those with coagulopathy or recent thrombolysis
- Arterial lines should not be used in delivery of medication

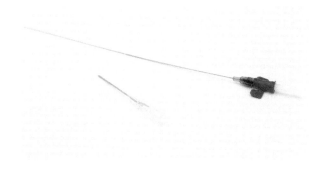

Urinary catheter

Description:
- Flexible plastic hollow tube which may be inserted through the urethra into the bladder, allowing drainage of urine
- Urinary catheters may be made of rubber, plastic, or silicone, and vary in diameter between 12Fr (4mm) and 30Fr (10mm)

Indication:
- Management of acute urinary retention, commonly secondary to prostate enlargement, urinary tract infections and constipation
- Accurate monitoring of fluid balance in critically ill patients such as those with sepsis, heart failure and acute kidney injury

Directions of use:
- Clean hands with soap and warm water and apply sterile gloves and appropriate PPE
- Open and prepare contents sterile catheter pack carefully, ensuring maintenance of sterile field
- Expose the patient appropriately, note patient should be supine, with bed at a comfortable height, placing absorbent pad underneath patient's genital area.
- Clean the genital area using gauze and saline
- Insert local anaesthetic gel from syringe into the urethral meatus, completely emptying 5ml syringe slowly
- Allow 3–5 minutes for gel to numb the area
- Gently insert catheter into the urethra (support the penis in a male patient and part the labia in a female)
- Advance catheter slowly, if resistance is met on repeated attempts, specialist urological input should be sought

- Once fully inserted, urine should begin to drain.
- Inflate balloon using 10ml sterile water containing syringe
- Once balloon is fully inflated, withdraw catheter gently until resistance is met and attach catheter bag securely
- Clean and dispose of equipment and allow patient to redress in privacy

Cautions and contraindications:
- Indwelling catheters can cause bladder spasms, haematuria, urethritis
- Catheters may stop draining and start bypassing urine if catheter becomes blocked
- Catheters predispose patients to urinary tract infection
- Take caution in catheterisation of elderly males, as patients with enlarged prostates may have technically difficult catheter insertions

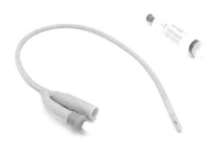

Intravenous cannulation kit

Description:

- Intravenous (IV) cannula consists of a hollow plastic tube, which surrounds the outer surface of a removable trocar needle, which is typically inserted into a superficial peripheral vein
- IV cannulae are available in various diameter sizes ranging from 26G (smallest) to 14G (biggest) which are colour coded
- Accompanying octopus attachments are single of multiple lumen extensions attached to the cannula
- Giving sets consist of a luer connector, hollow tubing, V-track controller, filter and drip chamber, to allow and control the rate of infusion of fluids into an intravenous cannula

Indication:

- Wide range of clinical applications, including drug administration, fluid resuscitation and transfusions of blood components
- An octopus attachment allows multiple intravenous therapies to be administered simultaneously
- For larger volumes, a giving set allows delivery of medications and fluids in a controlled manner

Directions of use:

- Wash hands and wear appropriate PPE
- Apply tourniquet proximally and observe/palpate for suitable vein
- Clean skin using an alcohol swab, allowing sufficient time for skin to dry
- Unsheath cannula and insert into vein at a shallow angle of 5–30 degrees

- Once flashback is seen, advance the cannula into vein and remove needle
- At this point, the cap can be attached to stop flow of blood
- Flush octopus with normal saline and attach to cannula
- Flush octopus and cannula with normal saline to ensure patency of vein, checking for pain or swelling around the cannula site
- Using adhesive stickers, secure cannula to skin
- Giving set can now be attached for delivery of intravenous therapies

Cautions and contraindication:
- Common complications include bleeding, haematoma, insertion-site infection, phlebitis and extravasation
- Relative contraindications to insertion include localised infection, phlebitis, sclerosed veins, burns or traumatic injury proximal to the insertion site and arteriovenous fistula in an extremity

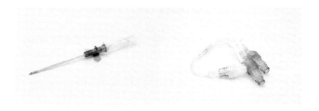

Intraosseous drill kit

Description:
- Intraosseous (IO) needle with accompanying powered insertion device
- Typically consists of handheld cordless drill and specialised needle with overlying non-collapsible metal catheter, with luer-lock attachment

Indication:
- Circulatory resuscitation in cases where peripheral vascular access is difficult to obtain
- IO access can be used for delivery of fluids and drugs
- Blood sampling may also be undertaken intraosseously
- Immediate vascular access can be obtained during cardiac arrest and in life-threatening systemic shock

Directions of use:
- Common sites of insertion include proximal tibia, distal tibia, distal femur, proximal humerus (adults), and superior iliac crest (children)
- Identify the insertion site, clean skin using alcohol swab allowing time to dry
- Advance drill and needle attachment at 90 degree angle into the bone gently, until give is felt as the needle enters the medullary space
- Unscrew the stylet from the needle and corresponding tubing
- Aspirate using syringe and flush using 0.9% saline flush, to confirm positioning
- Beware of extravasation
- Secure IO cannula to skin using adhesive and administer medications or infusion fluids

Cautions and contraindications:

- Contraindications to IO insertion include target bone fracture, localised infection or burn injury, inability to identify bony landmarks, recent IO access or attempt in last 48 hours and osteogenesis imperfecta
- Complications include extravasation injury, local haematoma, infection and rarely compartment syndrome and fat embolism
- Do not send IO specimens for blood gas analysis, as this will cause damage to the analysis machines
- In children, care must be taken to avoid insertion near growth plates

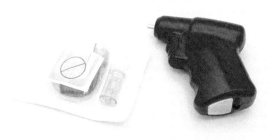

ECG machine

Description:
- Device used to record the electrical activity, rate and rhythm of the heart
- Typically consists of 12 electrodes attached to the limbs and chest connected to an analyser to detect and graphically display the electrical signals generated by the heart
- Commonly, traces can be printed on graph paper to be interpreted by clinical teams

Indication:
- Widespread use including assessment and diagnosis in symptoms such as palpitations, dizziness, cyanosis, chest pain, syncope, seizures and poisoning
- Symptoms or signs associated with heart disease including tachycardia, bradycardia and clinical conditions including hypothermia, murmur, shock, hypotension and hypertension

Directions of use:
- Appropriately expose patient and attach electrodes to correct electrode sites
- Ensure ECG machine is accurately calibrated
- Ask patient to remain still during the procedure
- Record and print out ECG trace

Cautions and contraindications:
- ECG analysis is simple, safe, non-invasive and causes no harm to patients
- Note that movement of the patient can cause distortion in electrical activity reading
- Furthermore, misplacement of ECG electrodes can cause inaccurate ECG traced, leading to inaccurate interpretation

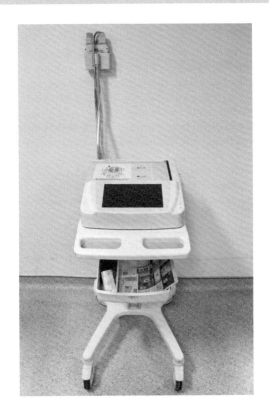

Defibrillator

Description:
- Advanced life support device which can monitor the electrical activity of the heart and deliver electrical shocks to aid restoration sinus rhythm in peri-arrest arrhythmias and cardiac arrest
- External defibrillator sets typically consists of a manual or automated defibrillator device along with connectible adhesive skin pads

Indication:
- Defibrillator and pads are essential in cardiac arrests, allowing for shocks to be delivered in ventricular fibrillation (VF) or pulseless ventricular tachycardia (VT)
- Defibrillators with a pacing function may also be used in peri-arrest arrhythmias including SVT and severe bradyarrhythmias to externally synchronise cardiac rhythm and maintain cardiac output

Directions of use:
- Only health care providers trained in Advanced Life Support (ALS) should attempt to use defibrillator devices
- Remove gel pads from packaging and attach one to the upper right chest, below the clavicle, and one pad to the left axillary area
- Turn on defibrillator and allow the rhythm to be read, halting chest compressions briefly as per ALS guidelines
- Some devices will be able to automatically detect shockable rhythms and shock, whereas others will require manual interpretation and shock delivery
- Defibrillator machines can also be used for transcutaneous pacing and electric cardioversion

Cautions and contraindications:

- Note that shocks should only be delivered by an automated defibrillator or an operator trained to interpret the electrical activity shown, as not all rhythms are shockable and inappropriate shocking may induce arrhythmias
- Defibrillation may pose a fire risk, therefore all open sources of oxygen must be intermittently removed from the patient during shocks
- Defibrillation may also cause accidental electrocution to health care providers, therefore all staff should keep a safe distance from the patient during shocks
- Defibrillation and chest compressions are not appropriate in those with do not attempt resuscitation (DNAR) orders.

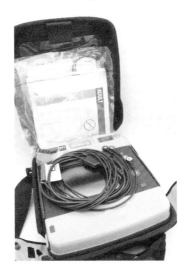

Cardiac monitor

Description:
- Medical device allowing for the continuous monitoring of the electrical activity of the heart
- The device will typically consist of 3 or 12 lead ECG leads attached to a monitor which can display heart traces in real time
- Cardiac monitoring is often paired with regular blood pressure, oxygen saturation and respiratory rate monitoring which may all be displayed on the same screen

Indication:
- Acutely unwell patients at risk of a cardiac event such as life-threatening arrhythmias or myocardial infarction
- Ambulatory cardiac monitoring may be indicated for outpatients under investigation for various cardiac conditions

Directions of use:
- Apply ECG electrodes to the patient and attach to monitor
- The process is similar to the ECG machine and defibrillator (see *ECG Machine* and *Defibrillator*)

Cautions and contraindications:
- Improper placement of electrodes may lead to false trace, causing diagnostic confusion
- Patient movement may also distort electrical activity

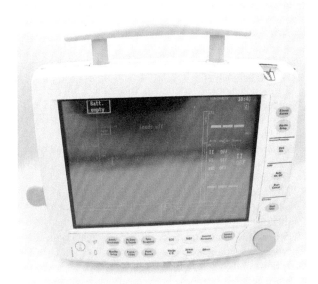

Venipuncture sample tubes

Description:
- Venous blood sample collection tubes used for the obtaining, storage and analysis of blood samples for various parameters
- Tubes, commonly referred to as Vacutainers, are typically under a vacuum to facilitate the drawing up of blood and may contain various additives to stabilise and preserve the blood sample for analysis
- Different blood tests require different additives and their tube caps are colour coded as such

Indications:
- Blood tests such as biochemistry, haematology and microbiology are helpful in aiding diagnostic and therapeutic decision making for clinicians
- See table of sample tubes for further information on types of vacutainers

Directions of use:
- Once access is established to vein, attach vacutainer or culture bottle to vacutainer needle and allow time for blood to flow
- Be careful to sufficiently fill bottles
- Be careful to fill bottles according to specified order of draw

Cautions and contraindications:
- Ensure to correctly label all samples
- To avoid cross-contamination of additives between tubes, blood must be drawn in a specific order
- Relative contraindications to venipuncture include localised oedema, burns, cellulitis, ipsilateral arm mastectomy or arteriovenous fistula

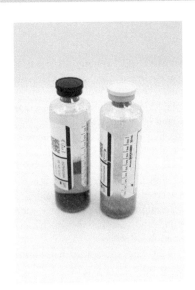

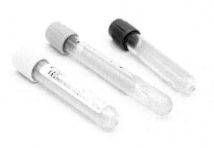

Central venous line

Description:
- Also known as a central venous catheter (CVC)
- Catheter placed directly into a large vein, allowing venous access
- Common placement includes internal jugular vein, subclavian vein or axillary vein
- The catheter may contain multiple lumens, allowing for delivery of multiple therapies

Indication:
- Patients with difficult peripheral venous access, who require regular venesection or delivery of medications intravenously
- Delivery of certain medications or fluids, such as chemotherapies and vasopressors, which can cause damage to peripheral veins
- Prolonged intravenous therapy, such as antibiotics or parenteral nutrition
- Certain treatments require a central line, such as haemodialysis, plasmapheresis and other forms of monitoring such as pulmonary artery catheterisation

Directions of use:
- The insertion of a central venous line should only be performed by trained health care professionals and its individual steps fall outside the scope of this book
- Clean the central line ports before and after each use with an alcohol swab
- Note in venesection the initial blood drawn into the syringe will not reflect the venous circulation, due to dilutional effects of previous medications and stasis of blood in the line

- Note that delivery of medications and venesection should both be followed with normal saline flush

Cautions and contraindications:
- Contraindications to insertion include distorted local anatomy (such as trauma), local infection, or thrombus within the intended vein
- Relative contraindications include coagulopathy, active bleeding from target vessel or proximal vascular injury
- Post-insertion complications include pain, hematoma, infection (both at insertion site or generalised bacteraemia), accidental arterial cannulation, vessel laceration or dissection, air embolism, thrombosis and pneumothorax requiring a possible chest tube

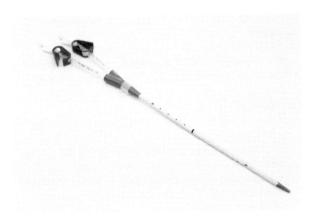

Disability

Pen torch

Description:
- Portable pocket light source used to examine pupils
- Size guide on side of torch for gauging pupillary size

Indication:
- Assessment of pupil size and light reflex
- Part of general ABCDE assessment, especially pertinent in cases of reduced GCS, head injury, suspected drug overdose

Directions of use:
- Assessment of pupil size – graded against size guide on pen (normal 2–5mm)
- Assessment of direct pupillary reflex – pupillary constriction on shining light in isolated eye
- Assessment of relative afferent pupillary reflex – assessed by swinging light torch method

Cautions and contraindications:
- No major complications of contraindications of note

DOI: 10.1201/9781003159179-5

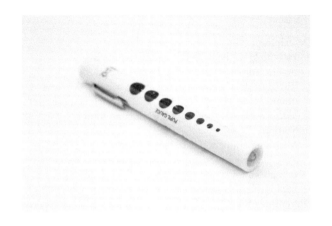

Glucose meter

Description:

- Handheld medical device used for point-of-care monitoring of capillary blood glucose level
- Two-part device consisting of lancet to prick skin and obtain blood sample; and glucometer which comprises of a disposable strip and digital readout monitor

Indication:

- Measurement of capillary blood glucose as part of ABCDE assessment, especially important in cases of reduced GCS and cases where blood glucose derangement is suspected

Directions of use:

- Load disposable strip into glucometer
- Clean fingerprick site with alcohol wipe
- Apply lancet to side of finger pulp and prick skin once
- Hold strip to blood sample until blood glucose reading appears
- Ensure skin prick site is cleaned and bleeding stops

Cautions and contraindications:

- Minor complications including bleeding, skin prick site infection

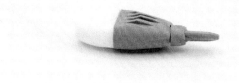

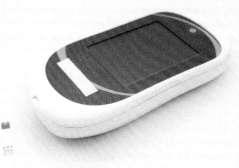

Exposure

Tympanic thermometer

Description:
- Handheld device equipped with heat-sensitive probe which is inserted into the external ear canal to measure patient's body temperature

Indication:
- Measure body temperature as part of general ABCDE assessment, especially important in causes of suspected pyrexia or hypothermia

Directions of use:
- Apply disposable cap to probe tip
- Insert probe into external ear canal
- Hold until temperature reading appears on display
- Dispose of probe cap

Cautions and contraindications:
- Avoid use in otitis interna/externa/local trauma/foreign body

DOI: 10.1201/9781003159179-6

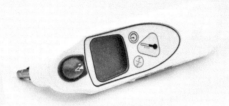

Trauma

Combat application tourniquet

Description:
- Cuff-like device placed around a limb and tightened to eliminate arterial flow past the device
- Commonly used tourniquets in the emergency setting include the combat application tourniquet (CAT) which consists of a securable strap and twistable windlass rod to ensure sufficient pressure

Indication:
- Major haemorrhage from extremity which cannot be controlled by direct pressure to the bleeding site

Directions of use:
- Insert bleeding limb through the tourniquet
- Place tourniquet proximal to bleeding site, as distal as possible, avoiding joints
- Pull self-adhering strap tight and fasten it
- Twist windlass rod until all arterial bleeding has stopped
- Lock windlass rod in windlass clip
- Record the time at which the tourniquet is applied

DOI: 10.1201/9781003159179-7

Cautions and contraindications:

- Distal ischaemic injury if applied for longer than 2 hours
- Reperfusion injury following tourniquet removal
- Inadequate tightening leading to continuation of haemorrhage

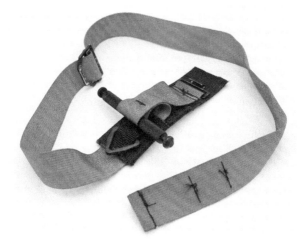

Cervical spine collar

Description:
- Rigid plastic brace which fits around the neck and is used to support the head and immobilise the cervical spine
- Multiple variations exist, but all generally comprise of a firm bi-valved shell secured by straps and lined by soft removable pads

Indication:
- Suspected cervical spine injury

Directions of use:
- Ensure patient in supine position
- Select appropriate size collar by measuring distance between patient's chin and root of the neck
- Restrict the motion of the neck by holding either side of the head (requires assistant)
- Slide the posterior part of the collar under the patient's neck
- Place the anterior part of the collar around the neck, ensuring the chin sits in the chin holder
- Secure the collar with the straps ensuring patient is able to open his or her mouth, but unable to flex the neck

Cautions and contraindications:
- Common complications include discomfort, skin breakdown and infection associated with long-term use
- Incorrect size selection or poor application can lead to unstable C-spine

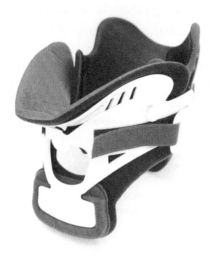

Pelvic binder

Description:
- Circumferential compression device secured around the pelvis in order to stabilise pelvic fractures and control bleeding
- Multiple variations exist, but all consist of a posterior low-friction sling and anterior strap or buckle

Indication:
- Suspected pelvic fracture

Directions of use:
- Identify appropriate landmarks, locating greater trochanters
- Slide device under the patient whilst restricting spinal motion and ensuring minimal motion of the pelvis by rotating patient laterally
- Rotate patient in the opposite direction and pull other end of device through
- Position patient back into supine position and secure the device anteriorly

Cautions and contraindications:
- Complications include incorrect placement and tissue breakdown associated with long-term use

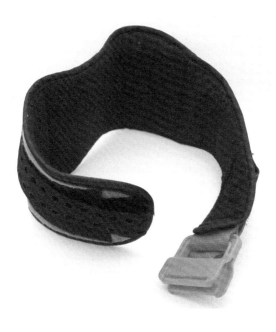

Trauma board

Description:
- Also known as "spine board" or "spinal board"
- Rigid board used for the immobilisation and transport of patients in emergency settings
- Often made of plastic and fitted with holes on either side to accommodate immobilisation straps

Indication:
- Suspected spinal injury

Directions of use:
- Before moving patient onto trauma board, ensure cervical spine is immobilised using C-spine collar (see *Cervical spine collar*)
- Ensure patient in supine position
- Place trauma board neck to patient and log roll away from board
- Slide board towards patient and log roll patient back onto ward
- Secure the patient onto the board with the immobilisation straps

Cautions and contraindications:
- Complications include inadequate immobilisation leading to lack of spinal support; pain and discomfort and pressure sore development following long-term use

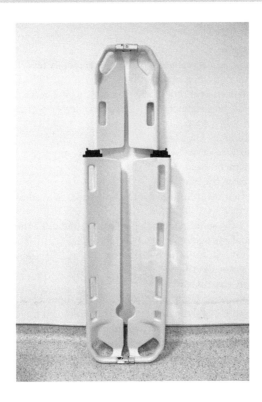

Traction splint

Description:
- Emergency device used to assist in temporary reduction and stabilisation of femoral fractures
- Variations exist, but largely consist of a ratchet traction device, heel stand, metal rod supports, leg support straps and ischial strap

Indication:
- Suspected or obvious midshaft femur fractures

Directions of use:
- Stabilise the injured leg
- Position the splint against the uninjured leg to adjust the length
- Place the splint under the patient's leg and place the ischial pad against the ischial tuberosity
- Adjust splint to length, then attach an ischial strap over the groin and thigh
- Apply the ankle hitch to the patient
- Apply gentle but firm traction until the injured leg length is approximately equal to the uninjured leg length
- Secure the remaining velcro straps around the leg
- Reassess neurovascular function

Cautions and contraindications:
- Common complications include local pressure sore from prolonged use
- Contraindications include use in ankle or foot fractures, or use in a partially amputated or severely damaged distal limb

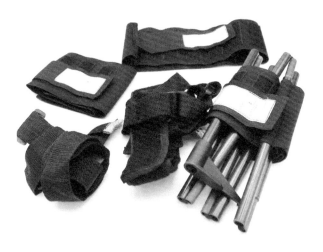

Ultrasound machine

Description:
- Ultrasound machine used for rapid bedside examination in trauma patients known as *focused assessment with sonography in trauma* (commonly abbreviated as FAST scan)

Indication:
- Blunt and/or penetrating abdominal and/or thoracic trauma
- Undifferentiated shock and/or hypotension

Directions of use:
- 2–5 MHz curvilinear (or abdominal) probe is typically used
- Four windows are used to viewed 10 structures in sequence
- Cardiac window – used to view pericardium and heart chambers
- Right upper quadrant – used to view hepatorenal recess, liver tip and lower right thorax
- Left upper quadrant – used to view subphrenic space, splenorenal recess, spleen tip and lower left thorax
- Pelvic window – used to view rectovesical pouch (in males), or rectouterine pouch (in females)

Cautions and contraindications:
- There are no absolute contraindications to performing a FAST scan, however, a FAST scan should not delay resuscitation during ATLS management

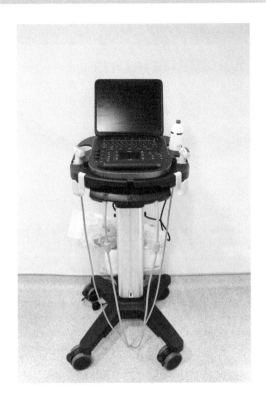

Miscellaneous

Alcohol swab/chloraprep

Description:
- Small rectangular swab containing high concentrations of alcohol, usually 70%
- Chloraprep is an antiseptic solution containing both 70% alcohol and 2% chlorhexidine

Indications:
- Commonly used to disinfect small areas of skin in procedures such as peripheral cannulation and venesection
- Chloraprep solution is commonly applied to skin in sterilisation in larger procedures such as drain insertion or lumbar puncture

Directions of use:
- Using a gloved hand, take a swab or chloraprep applicator and thoroughly clean the target area
- Start from the cleanest area, usually the procedure site and proceed in a concentric fashion to the least clean area
- Allow time for solution to dry before commencing procedure

DOI: 10.1201/9781003159179-8

Cautions and contraindications:
- Alcohol swabs can cause local irritation, allergic reactions and dry skin, especially on repeated use
- Note alcohol is flammable and care must be taken to allow the solution to dry
- Chloraprep can also cause local irritation and allergic reaction

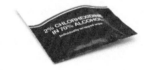

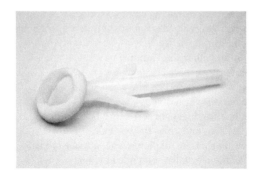

Syringe

Description:
- Plastic cylindrical tube and plunger equipped with a nozzle at the distal end, allowing for delivery and suction of liquids and medications
- Syringes come in various volumes (typically indicated in millilitres) and have a multitude of uses
- Some syringes in clinical settings will have a luer lock system to allow for easy connection to medical equipment such as central lines and octopus attachments

Indication:
- Syringes are used in a multitude of clinical settings, including delivery of medication and fluids
- Syringes may also be used to remove body fluids

Directions of use:
- Pull plunger to suction liquid into the syringe, push plunger to deliver liquid from the syringe
- Always ensure the correct medication and dose is selected before drawing up into syringe
- When drawing up medications, ensure no air bubbles remain in the syringe

Cautions and contraindications:
- Syringes are generally safe to use
- Always use appropriate PPE when administering medications via syringe
- Ensure all syringes are correctly labelled with medications and doses they contain
- Be aware that not all plungers are attached to the syringe and liquid may fall out if pulled too far

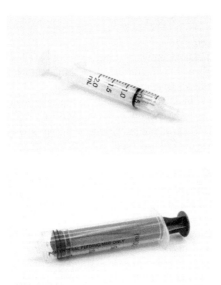

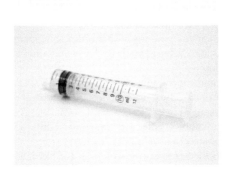

Hypodermic needle

Description:
- Thin, hollow metal tube equipped with bevelled sharp tip to allow for penetration of the skin and injection or extraction of substances from the body
- The proximal end of the needle is typically coated in plastic and may be connected to a syringe
- Needles are available in various sizes (typically described as Gauge or "G") and types

Indication:
- Needles are used in many medical procedures such as aspiration, injection and even biopsy
- Needles can be used to puncture and gain access to many tissues, such as vessels or skin
- Needles are also used to draw up medications and fluids

Directions of use:
- Variable depending on indication
- Select correct gauge and type of needle for intended procedure
- Wear appropriate PPE
- Disinfect skin intended for injection
- Ensure careful handling of sharps throughout procedure and dispose of sharps safely in sharps container following procedure

Cautions and contraindications:
- Needles can cause damage to local structures and bleeding upon insertion
- Always handle needles with caution and dispose of them appropriately to avoid sharps injuries
- Care should be taken in coagulopathy and bleeding disorders

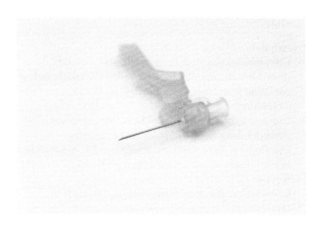

Gloves

Description:

- Disposable gloves used during medical or surgical procedures and examinations, covering the hands and providing protection to both patient and healthcare professional
- Gloves are commonly made of latex, but may also be made of rubber, polyvinyl chloride, or neoprene
- Examination glove sizes vary from XS to XL, meanwhile sterile surgical gloves are sized from 5.5 to 8.5

Indication:

- Examination gloves are commonly used in medical examinations, to prevent cross-contamination of patients and medical professionals
- Sterile surgical gloves are used in invasive medical procedures and surgery, both of which require sterile or aseptic conditions

Directions of use:

- Select appropriate size and type of glove for procedure to be undertaken
- Ensure thorough handwashing before gloving
- Examination gloves are typically interchangeable between left and right hands
- Surgical gloves have corresponding left and right hand and care must be taken to maintain aseptic technique during gloving

Cautions and contraindications:

- Commonly, some people may experience irritation and allergy to certain materials of glove

- Gloves may also perforate or split during procedures, reducing their effectiveness in preventing cross-contamination
- Double gloving may be advised in certain procedures where risk of infectious transmission is high

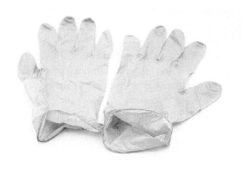

Personal protective equipment

Description:
- Protective garments and equipment used during times of patient contact in order to protect against transmission of infections and other risks of health and safety
- Commonly used PPE include gloves (see *Gloves*), aprons/gowns, masks and eye protection

Indication:
- Risk of exposure to blood, bodily fluids, secretions or excretions or when handling contaminated equipment
- Risk of pathogens spread by airborne route, e.g. measles, tuberculosis, chickenpox
- When performing aerosol generating procedures in patients with respiratory tract infections, e.g. COVID-19 or influenza
- Always follow local PPE guidelines and patient-specific policies

Directions of use:
- Disposable items of PPE should never be re-used and should be disposed of appropriately
- All items of PPE must be changed between patients
- Respirator masks may require "fit testing" before first use to ensure correct fit and functioning

Cautions and contraindications:
- PPE is generally safe to use
- Skin irritation may occur following prolonged use of PPE, especially tight-fitting masks

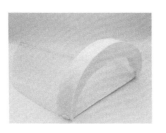

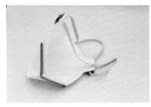

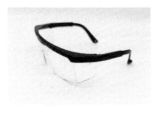

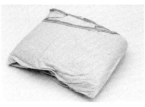

Lubricant

Description:
- Water-based soluble substance used to provide lubrication for multiple medical and surgical procedures and to lessen patient discomfort
- Typically contained in small sachets
- Lubricants may contain antiseptic or analgesic agents

Indication:
- Internal manual examinations such as vaginal or rectal examination
- Various invasive procedures such as urinary catheter insertion, endoscopy, endotracheal intubation etc.

Directions of use:
- Select appropriate lubricant for procedure
- Apply to surgical instrument in use or gloved hand, ensuring adequate coverage
- Clean of lubricant from surface following procedure

Cautions and contraindications:
- Lubricants are generally safe to use and poses minimal risk to both patients and health care professionals

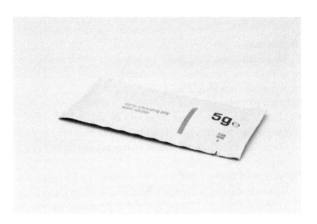

Universal specimen container

Description:
- Seal tight screw top plastic container in which biological samples may be stored and transported
- Available in multiple sizes

Indication:
- Microbiological analysis, especially of pus and other body specimens, for the presence of infectious agents
- Histopathological sampling of tissues especially in suspected cases of cancer

Directions of use:
- Wear appropriate PPE when handling samples
- Ensure container is properly sealed following sampling
- Correctly label sample with patient and sample details

Cautions and contraindications:
- No major safety considerations

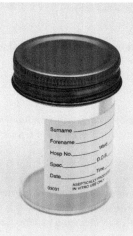

Specimen collection swab

Description:

- Absorbent cotton swab mounted on a plastic rod to enable the swabbing of various body parts on orifices
- Swab container tube may contain transport media or preservatives to aid subsequent analysis

Indication:

- Collection of biological samples for analysis by microbiology, virology, cytology or serology

Directions of use:

- Wear appropriate PPE when collecting samples
- Select appropriate swab and container for procedure
- Ensure swab only touches intended specimen for collection to avoid contamination
- Label swab with specimen and patient details following collection

Cautions and contraindications:

- No major safety concerns

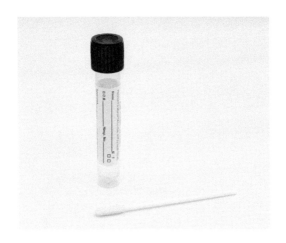

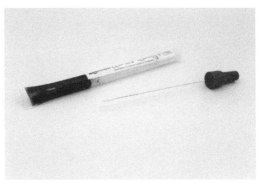

Section II

Specialty equipment

Cardiology

Echocardiography ultrasound machine

Description:
- Ultrasound machine equipped with Doppler capabilities to allow real-time imaging of the structure and dynamic function of the heart
- Echocardiography may be performed either via transthoracic or transoesophageal approach, with the latter requiring sedation

Indication:
- Non-invasive, real-time imaging of cardiac structures such as valves, ventricles, atria and pericardium in variety of cardiac pathologies
- Common presentations requiring echocardiography include palpitations, syncope, pre-syncope, newly diagnosed bundle branch blocks, arrhythmias, acute coronary syndrome, exertional shortness of breath and evaluation of pulmonary hypertension

DOI: 10.1201/9781003159179-10

Directions of use:

- The following section will describe the steps in transthoracic echocardiography
- Position the patient in the lateral position
- Ensure probe has sufficient ultrasound gel applied to allow for adequate contact with the skin
- Place the probe along the predefined positions along the chest to allow visualisation of the following views: parasternal long axis, parasternal short axis, apical four-chamber and subxiphoid

Cautions and contraindications:

- Transthoracic echocardiography is safe and non-invasive
- Transoesophageal echocardiography may be associated with esophageal perforation or bleeding

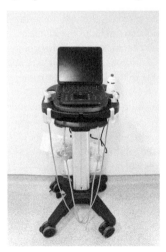

Gastroenterology

Nasogastric tube

Description:

- Flexible hollow rubber or plastic tube, which is inserted through the nose to pass through the posterior oropharynx, down the esophagus and into the stomach
- Allows for the decompression of the stomach, or the controlled nutrition or delivery of medications in patients who are unable to tolerate an oral intake

Indication:

- Multiple indications, but commonly include the following
- Small bowel obstruction
- Unsafe swallow following stroke or any other local neurological or anatomical dysfunction
- ITU patients under sedation

Directions of use:

- Gather essential equipment, including correct size NG tube, lubricant and PPE

DOI: 10.1201/9781003159179-11

- Measure the estimated length required to pass into the stomach by looping the NG tube around the patient's ear and placing the tip over the xiphoid process
- Warn the patient of some potential discomfort on insertion
- Gently pass the lubricated NG tube along the floor of the nose, directed towards the back of the throat
- As the tube is further advanced, ask the patient to swallow to aid the passage of the NG down the oesophagus
- If firm resistance is met, withdraw slightly and gently attempt reinsertion
- The NG tube should typically reach about 55cm of insertion in an adult
- Once in place, ensure secured to nose with tape
- Aspiration must be obtained showing acidic pH, otherwise positioning should be confirmed using chest X-ray

Cautions and contraindications:

- Common complications include discomfort, sinusitis or epistaxis
- Accidental placement into the airway may occur, highlighting need to confirm position via pH strip or X-ray before use
- Long-term NG placement may lead to localised erosion of nasal ala, nasal cavity and nasopharynx
- Contraindications include significant facial trauma or base of skull fractures
- Oesophageal trauma may also be a relative contraindication in certain cases

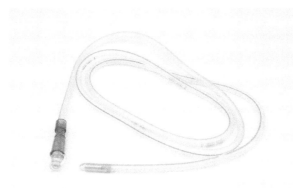

Paracentesis kit

Description
- Hollow catheter inserted into abdomen to allow sampling or drainage of ascitic fluid
- Prepackaged paracentesis kits are available which typically comprise of a scalpel, paracentesis catheter with removable introducer needle, syringe and drainage bag

Indication:
- Suspicion of spontaneous bacterial peritonitis
- New onset ascites of unknown cause
- Tense Ascites causing discomfort or respiratory distress
- Recurrent ascites refractory to diuretic treatment

Directions of use:
- Gather equipment and wear appropriate PPE
- Position patient comfortably lying supine
- Use bedside ultrasound to correctly identify appropriate area for drain insertion (see *Ultrasound Machine*)
- Prep skin with antiseptic solution (see *Antiseptic Solution*) and administer local anaesthetic to area
- Use scalpel to make small skin incision overlying intended site of drain insertion
- Advance catheter needle through the skin and underlying soft tissue until give is felt, signalling the peritoneum has been entered
- Advance the catheter while removing the introducer needle
- Secure the catheter and attach drainage bag
- Sampling from catheter may now be performed

Cautions and contraindications:

- Relative contraindications coagulopathy, thrombocytopenia, local skin infection, and pregnancy
- Possible complications include persistent ascitic leak, haematoma or bleeding, infection and rarely perforation of intra-abdominal viscera
- Caution should be taken with large volume (above 5L of ascites) drainage and Human Albumin Solution (HAS) should be administered to avoid hypotension

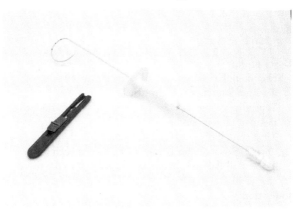

Neurology

Tendon hammer

Description:
- Hammer-like instrument, allowing for the eliciting of deep tendon reflexes when struck
- Typically consist of rubberised weighted head attached to metal or plastic handle
- Most commonly used tendon hammers in the UK are the Queens Square reflex hammers, but others such as the Taylor and Babinski hammer are also used in the rest of the world

Indication:
- Assessing the amplitude of deep tendon reflexes including those of the biceps (C5–C6), triceps (C7–C8), brachioradialis (C5–C6), patella (L2–L4) and ankle (S1)
- Forms a key component of the general neurological examination

Directions of use:
- Position the patient so that the joint around which the reflex is tested is fully relaxed

DOI: 10.1201/9781003159179-12

- In one swift arc, swing the hammer and strike directly onto corresponding area to elicit reflex
- Observe the proximal muscle group for contraction
- Systematically work through all of the deep tendon reflexes comparing like for like
- Distraction techniques, such as the Jendrassik maneuver, may be used to help relaxation of the targeted joint

Cautions and contraindications:

- Tendon hammers are generally safe to use with no safety concerns

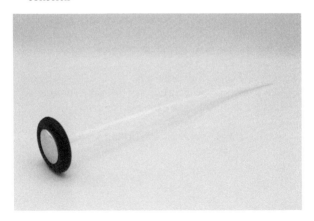

Neurotip

Description:
- Sterile single use neurological examination pins used for the testing of pain sensation

Indication:
- Used to test for pain sensation in neurological examination

Directions of use:
- Gently apply force to skin of dermatomal area being tested
- Note patient's ability to detect character and amplitude of sensation
- Systematically work through dermatomal areas comparing like for like

Cautions and contraindications:
- Take caution when applying force through neurotip, excessive force can cause excessive pain and puncture of skin
- Avoid use in areas of local skin infection

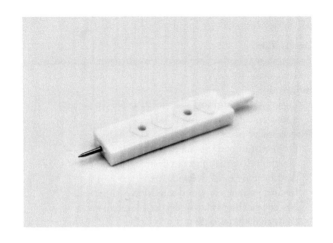

Cotton bud

Description:
- Simple soft cotton swab used for testing of light touch sensation

Indication:
- Light touch sensation assessment as part of general neurological examination

Directions of use:
- Form cotton bud into a fine cotton tip
- Touch cotton tip lightly to desired dermatome or nerve distribution being assessed
- Record patient's reported sensation
- Systematically work through dermatomal areas comparing like for like

Cautions and contraindications:
- Cotton buds are safe to use

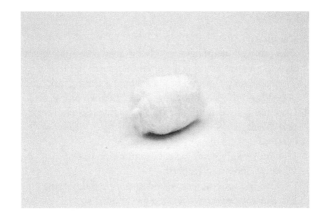

Tuning fork

Description:
- Two-pronged metal device with flattened base that, when struck, vibrates at a specific pitch (measured in Hz)
- The frequency of sound produced by the tuning fork depends on the length and weight of the two prongs
- Commonly used tuning forks in medicine include 128Hz and 512Hz

Indication:
- Used in sensory neurological examination to test vibration sensation (128Hz)
- Used to test for conductive and sensorineural hearing loss in Rinne's and Webber's tests (512Hz)

Sensory vibration test:
- Select 128Hz tuning fork
- Strike tuning fork to elicit vibration and sound
- Place vibrating tuning fork onto specific part of the body and abruptly stop vibration by grasping both prongs of the fork
- Note if patient is able to detect the stop in vibration

Rinne's and Webbers test:
- Webers test: Strike tuning fork to elicit vibration at 512Hz, place at the midline on top of the forehead; sound will lateralise away from the affected ear
- Rinnes: Strike tuning fork to elicit vibration, place the base of the tuning fork on the mastoid bone. Once the patient is no longer able to hear the note via bone conduction, place the tuning fork near the entrance to the auditory canal. In normal hearing, air conduction

will be greater than bone conduction. Sensorineural deficit is present if bone conduction is worse than air conduction.

Cautions and contraindications:
* Tuning forks are safe to use

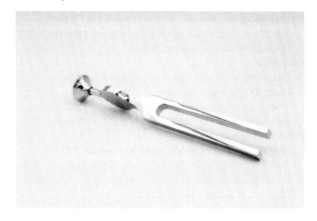

Lumbar puncture kit

Description:
- Spinal needle allowing for the sampling of cerebrospinal fluid (CSF) from the subarachnoid space of the lumbar spine
- Prepackaged lumbar puncture kits typically contain a spinal needle with stylet, CSF collection vials and manometer with three-way valve

Indication:
- Diagnosis of meningitis/encephalitis, subarachnoid haemorrhage and other neurological disorders
- Therapeutic intrathecal administration of medications such as anaesthetics, antibiotics and chemotherapy agents

Directions of use:
- Prepare all equipment and wear appropriate PPE
- Position patient in left lateral position with knees to chest
- Anatomical site of L4 identified by taking the midline of the highest points of both iliac crests
- Palpate above and below for the space between L3/4 and L4/5 and mark area of needle insertion
- Clean are with antiseptic solution
- Using aseptic technique, anaesthetise the overlying skin
- Insert the needle with stylet smoothly between the L3/4 or L4/5 interspace until a "pop" is felt, indicating passing through the ligamentum flavum
- After passing the ligamentum flavum, slowly advance the needle, removing the stylet to check for CSF drainage
- Opening pressures should be recorded using the manometer and CSF should be sent for microbiological and biochemical analysis

Cautions and contraindications:

- Contraindications include raised intracranial pressure (ICP), local skin infection, vertebral trauma, low platelet count and coagulopathy
- Complications include headache, bleeding/haematoma, infection, back pain
- A serious but rare complication is cerebral herniation, highlighting the importance to perform a CT head before the procedure to rule out raised ICP

Respiratory medicine

Non-invasive ventilation

Description:
- Ventilatory support machine used for the delivery of
  Continuous Positive Airway Pressure (CPAP) or Bilevel
  Positive Airway Pressure Support (BiPAP), which allows
  delivery of oxygen and improved ventilation without
  invasive intubation
- The circuit typically consists of a tight-fitting mask,
  tubing and pump with adjustable pressure settings

Indication:
- CPAP is commonly indicated in conditions causing type
  1 respiratory failure, such as pulmonary oedema and
  acute respiratory distress syndrome, severe pneumonia or
  COVID pneumonitis
- BiPAP is commonly indicated in type 2 respiratory failure
  commonly seen in COPD exacerbation and opiate toxicity

Directions of use:
- Ensure face mask is fitted correctly and required pressure(s)
  are set on NIV machine

DOI: 10.1201/9781003159179-13

- Check machine reading for pressure leak to assess efficacy
- Typically, patients on NIV will require monitoring through regular arterial blood gasses to check for adequate ventilation and oxygenation

Cautions and contraindications:

- Complications include barotrauma leading to pneumothorax, pneumomediastinum and surgical emphysema
- Long-term use of NIV face mask can also lead to facial pressure sores
- Absolute contraindications include facial injury or recent upper airway surgery, uncontrolled vomiting/upper GI bleeding
- Contraindications (requiring consideration of intubation) include airway obstruction/unstable airway, life threatening hypoxaemia, confusion/delirium, bowel obstruction, severe co-morbidity, excess secretions
- NIV should be used with caution in the presence of a pneumothorax. Most patients should have intercostal drain insertion prior to NIV.

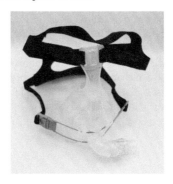

High flow nasal cannulae

Description:
- Nasal cannulae providing oxygen therapy at increased flow rates (up to 60L/min) for patients, generally in type 1 respiratory failure
- Increased rates of flow dilate the upper airways, allowing for reduced resistance and increased ventilation
- High flow nasal cannulae allow for oxygen heating and humidification, providing greater comfort

Indication:
- Type 1 respiratory failure, including pneumonia and pulmonary oedema
- Pre- and post-extubation oxygenation
- Obstructive sleep apnoea
- Patients unsuitable for intubation

Directions of use:
- See *Nasal Cannulae* for detailed instructions
- Humidification and heating may be controlled and optimised to the patient's needs

Cautions and contraindications:
- Patients with facial injuries may not tolerate nasal cannulae
- Patients with blockages of the nasal canals will be unable to receive oxygen therapy using this method
- Prolonged use of nasal cannulae may lead to local nasal skin breakdown and ulceration

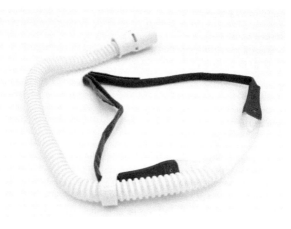

Peak flow meter

Description:
- Reusable hand-held device used to measure the peak expiratory flow rate of patients
- Typically consists of a cylindrical plastic device with a slidable indicator on the side and a single-use attachable mouthpiece

Indication:
- Evaluation of asthma severity
- Monitor response to asthma treatment

Directions of use:
- Ensure that the slidable indicator is reset to zero before use
- Whilst sitting up or standing, take a deep breath
- Form a tight seal around the mouthpiece and produce a single, fast and forceful breath out
- Repeat the process 3–4 times and record the highest reading

Cautions and contraindications:
- Peak flow readings should not be undertaken in patients who are severely short of breath with respiratory distress as it may delay management

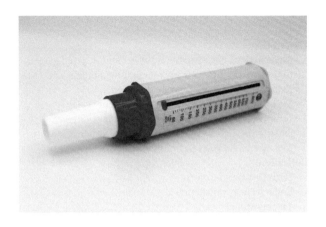

Humidifier

Description:
- Medical device used to humidify air and inspired gases to prevent drying of airway mucosal membranes and to reduce the build-up of mucus secretions
- Various types of humidification exist, but typically comprises of a high concentration of air or oxygen passing through a water circuit, which is then connected to a facemask or nasal cannulae

Indication:
- High flow nasal oxygen
- Endotracheal ventilation
- Tracheostomy
- Airway secretion management

Directions of use:
- Fill required volume of distilled water into reservoir bottle
- Attach air or oxygen supply to reservoir bottle
- Connect downstream oxygen delivery equipment, e.g. facemask or nasal cannula
- Ensure oxygen flow set to correct rate

Cautions and contraindications:
- Humidifiers are contraindicated in patients with thick, copious or bloody secretions

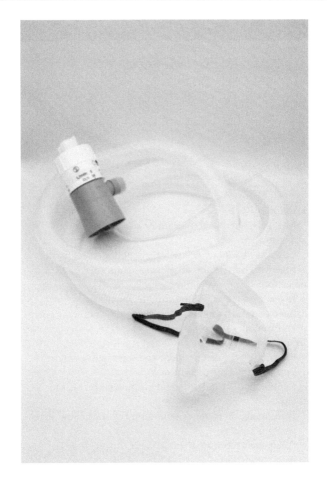

General surgery

Proctoscope

Description:
- Medical device used to examine the anal cavity and rectum
- Consists of a short, straight, rigid, hollow, clear plastic tube with handle and attachable light source

Indication:
- Inspection for anorectal disease, such as haemorrhoids, anal fissures, proctitis, anorectal polyps and tumours

Directions of use:
- Explain procedure to patient and warn of discomfort
- Ensure chaperone present
- Position patient in left lateral position with knees to chest
- Perform digital rectal examination before attempting to pass proctoscope
- Adequately lubricate the outside of the proctoscope before insertion

DOI: 10.1201/9781003159179-14

- Gently insert proctoscope into rectum and inspect anorectal passage systematically
- Ensure no immediate complications such as bleeding upon removal of scope

Cautions and contraindications:

- Complications include discomfort post examination, tearing of perianal skin or mucosa and more rarely infection post-procedure
- Anal stenosis or severe pain on digital rectal examination is a contraindication to passage of proctoscope
- Proctoscopy should not be performed on an imperforate anus

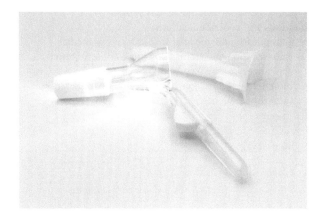

Stoma bag

Description:
- Plastic bag attached to abdominal stoma site to allow collection of waste from the digestive tract
- Consists of a flange which adheres to the skin and a detachable pouch which carries the waste and may be emptied at regular intervals

Indication:
- Patients requiring colostomy or ileostomy commonly due to inflammatory bowel disease, diverticulitis or colorectal cancer

Directions of use:
- The application, removal and emptying of the stoma bags is taught by and carried out by specialist stoma nurses and is beyond the scope of this book

Cautions and contraindications:
- Complications associated with stoma bags include skin irritation and stoma leaks due to ill-fitting stoma appliance
- Stoma site bleeding may rarely occur due to irritation from the stoma bag

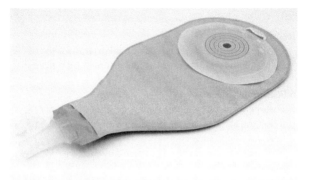

Drain bag

Description:
- Clear plastic bag attached to surgical drain used to collect fluid from drain site and measure drain output
- Available in multiple sizes

Indication:
- Postoperative surgical site fluid drainage, commonly following abdominal, thoracic, breast, orthopaedic and head and neck surgery
- Drainage of gastric contents when attached to nasogastric tube

Directions of use:
- The selection and attachment of drainage bag is commonly performed intraoperatively by the operating surgeon
- Assessment of drainage bags on the ward consists of output measurement and assessment of contents
- The decision to remove surgical drains following reduction or cessation of output is made by the operating surgeon

Cautions and contraindications:
- Complications of surgical drains include local pain, drain site infection, obstruction of drain and complications associated with drain removal

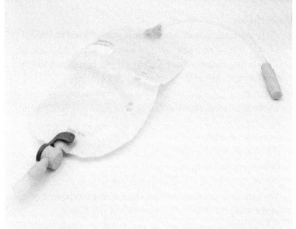

Redivac drain bottle

Description:
- Active vacuum assisted drainage system used in the postoperative management of surgical site fluid drainage
- The bottle comprises of a clear plastic container, drain connection site and vacuum indicator nozzle

Indication:
- Prevent postoperative collection of fluid following major surgery

Directions of use:
- The drain will be connected intraoperatively by the operating surgeon
- When reviewing the drain postoperatively, ensure that the circuit is connected and the vacuum indicator nozzle is showing an intact vacuum within the bottle
- The decision to remove the drain will be made by the operating surgeon

Cautions and contraindications:
- Complications include disconnection of the drain or vacuum, blockage of the drain, drain site infection and complications associated with drain removal

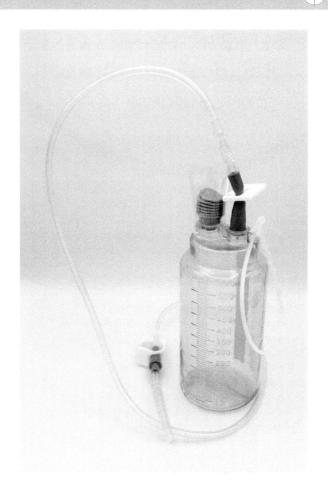

Ear, nose and throat (ENT) surgery

Tongue depressor

Description:
- Wooden or metal spatula used to push the tongue inferiorly to allow inspection of the buccal cavity and oropharynx

Indication:
- Suspected oral or oropharyngeal pathology, e.g. tonsillitis, quinsy, ingested foreign body
- To inspect for oropharyngeal blood in the case of epistaxis

Directions of use:
- Warn the patient that procedure may be uncomfortable
- Ask patient to open mouth as wide as possible
- Place tongue depressor along middle of the tongue and firmly push the tongue down
- Inspect the uvula, tonsillar tissue, palatal folds and posterior pharyngeal wall
- Dispose of tongue depressor after use

DOI: 10.1201/9781003159179-15

Cautions and contraindications:

- Tongue depressors are generally safe to use

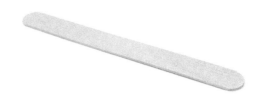

Otoscope

Description:
- Medical device used to inspect the tympanic membrane and external ear canal
- Commonly comprise of a handle and a head which is equipped with an internal light source and low-power magnifying lens
- Distal part of head enables attachment of disposable plastic ear speculum

Indication:
- Suspected outer or middle ear pathology, e.g. otitis externa, otitis media, foreign bodies, local trauma

Directions of use:
- Apply appropriate size disposable speculum to head (usually adult or paediatric size)
- Turn on internal light source
- Straighten ear canal by gently pulling pinna superoposteriorly
- Insert ear speculum part of otoscope into ear canal whilst placing the index finger or little finger against the head to avoid sudden movement of the otoscope
- Inspect the ear through the lens systematically
- Dispose of ear speculum

Cautions and contraindications:
- Local trauma may be caused in cases of forceful examination

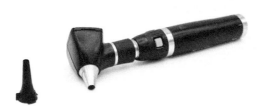

Flexible nasendoscope

Description:
- Narrow fiberoptic flexible telescope equipped with a light source which is passed through the nostril and allows the inspection of the upper aerodigestive tract
- Typically available in adult and paediatric sizes

Indication:
- Suspected upper aerodigestive pathology, e.g. ingested foreign body, sinusitis, nasal polyposis, malignancy, vocal cord dysfunction

Directions of use:
- Explain procedure to patient and warn it may be uncomfortable
- Sit patient upright and rest head against bed or wall
- Apply topical decongestant/anaesthetic spray into nostril
- Select appropriately sized nasendoscope for procedure
- Attach light source
- Lubricate tip of nasendoscope
- Gently pass nasendoscope into selected nostril
- Move and inspect along upper aerodigestive tract systematically
- Clean scope according to local policy once finished

Cautions and contraindications:
- Relative contraindications include epiglottis as nasendoscopy by inexperienced personnel may lead to laryngospasm and airway obstruction
- Nasendoscopy may rarely cause local trauma and bleeding

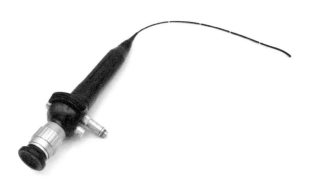

Silver nitrate cautery stick

Description:
- Wooden or plastic stick whose tip is covered in silver nitrate, used to chemically cauterise skin and mucous membrane in order to achieve localised haemostasis or destroy unwanted tissue

Indication:
- Haemostasis in anterior epistaxis or prevention of recurrent anterior epistaxis
- Cautery of skin tags, warts, and overproduction of granulation tissue

Directions of use:
- In case of epistaxis, apply directly to observed bleeding point under direct vision for few seconds using gentle rolling motion
- Stop application once bleeding stops and surrounding tissue seen to coagulate

Cautions and contraindications:
- Avoid bilateral cautery of nasal septum as this can lead to nasal septal necrosis
- Silver nitrate is corrosive to both skin and clothing so care should be taken to avoid unnecessary contact

Anterior nasal pack

Description:
- Intranasal haemostatic device used in the management of persistent epistaxis
- Key components include an absorbent nasal tampon with a string attached to aid subsequent retrieval
- May contain inflatable inner tube to aid compression of local bleeding vessels
- Common types include Rapid Rhino® and Merocel®

Indication:
- Epistaxis which has not stopped despite first aid measures or direct therapy to the bleeding point

Directions of use:
- Lubricate pack before insertion
- With non-dominant hand, push tip of nose up to reveal nostrils
- With dominant hand, insert pack horizontally, aiming for same vertical plane as ear lobe
- If inflatable inner tube present, inflate tube with 10–20ml of air using syringe
- Inspect for bleeding cessation following insertion

Cautions and contraindications:
- Posterior bleeding may still occur despite adequate anterior packing
- Prolonged nasal packing may lead to tissue breakdown due to direct pressure as well as local infection

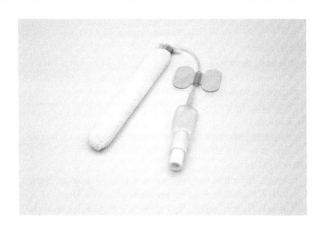

Nasal speculum

Description:
- Medical device used to inspect the anterior nasal cavity
- Consist of two flattened metal blades connected by a curved handle
- Available in both adult and paediatric sizes

Indication:
- Suspected anterior nasal cavity pathology, e.g. epistaxis, foreign bodies, rhinitis, trauma

Directions of use:
- Elevate the tip of the nose with the non-dominant hand
- With the dominant hand press the prongs of the speculum together to allow them to be placed within the nostril
- Reduce grip on the prongs to allow the blades to open further
- Inspect each nostril systematically

Cautions and contraindications:
- Nasal specula are generally safe to use
- May cause local trauma if used inappropriately

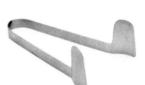

Headlight

Description:
- Wearable light source allowing for hands-free illumination of specific area of examination or surgical field
- Typically consists of adjustable headband, power source and light source

Indication:
- Examination or operation of body cavities with poor direct illumination, such as the oropharynx or deep neck spaces

Directions of use:
- Ensure power source fully charged before use
- Adjust headband accordingly
- Turn on light source and focus on area of interest

Cautions and contraindications:
- None

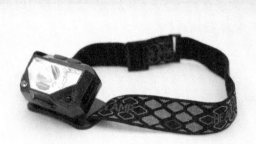

Urology

Urine sample collection pot

Description:
- Sterile plastic screw-top container used for the collection and laboratory processing of urine samples

Indication:
- Diagnosis and evaluation of urinary tract infections (UTIs) and sexually transmitted infections (STIs)
- Evaluation of renal function

Directions of use:
- Ensure pot correctly labelled with patient details
- Ask patient to give urine sample
- Ensure lid screwed shut before sending off for processing

Cautions and contraindications:
- When handling any body fluids ensure appropriate use of PPE to avoid contact and minimise potential infection risk

DOI: 10.1201/9781003159179-16

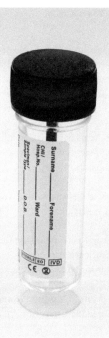

Three-way irrigation catheter

Description:
- Large diameter indwelling urinary catheter used for the washout and continuous irrigation of the bladder
- Comprises of three lumens used for urinary drainage, bladder irrigation and balloon inflation
- Irrigation lumen is connected to irrigation fluid

Indication:
- Removal of bladder debris or blood clot following haematuria
- Following urological surgery to prevent formation of blood clots

Directions of use:
- Please see *Urinary catheter* on steps of insertion
- Following catheter insertion, attach irrigation fluid bags to catheter
- Monitor drainage bag to ensure adequate urinary drainage

Cautions and contraindications:
- See *Urinary catheter* for complications associated with catheters
- Transurethral resection (TUR) syndrome may rarely occur as a result of bladder irrigation following transurethral surgery

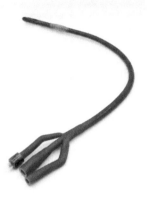

Bladder tip syringe

Description:
- Syringe equipped with a specialised tip allowing for the connection with a urinary catheter
- Used for the administration of fluid into the bladder for washout

Indication:
- Blocked catheter
- Significant urinary sediment or clots

Directions of use:
- Draw up 50ml normal saline into bladder tip syringe
- Attach syringe to urinary outflow lumen of catheter
- Push 50ml saline through catheter warning patient beforehand it may feel uncomfortable
- Aspirate 50ml saline from the catheter and discard
- Repeat process until aspirate is clear of sediment or clots

Cautions and contraindications:
- Bladder washout should be avoided in cases of autonomic dysreflexia as it could exacerbate symptoms
- Rarely bladder washouts may cause epithelial damage to the bladder

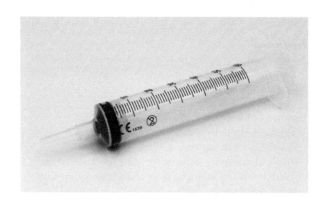

Bladder scanner

Description:
- Non-invasive portable ultrasound device used to assess the volume of retained urine in the bladder

Indication:
- Suspected cases of urinary retention

Directions of use:
- Explain procedure to patient
- Position patient supine
- Apply ultrasound conductive gel over lower abdomen
- Turn on bladder scan and place transducer 2–3cm over pubic symphysis
- Hold transducer in position until scan is done results appear on display
- Clean gel from transducer and patient's abdomen

Cautions and contraindications:
- Relative contraindications include pregnancy and open wounds in the suprapubic region

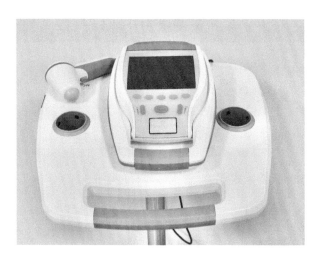

Musculoskeletal medicine

Graduated compression stockings

Description:
- Elastic stockings with gradually decreasing pressure gradient up the garment to ensure unilateral venous blood flow to the heart and to prevent venous pooling
- Compression stockings may vary in size and degrees of compression

Indication:
- Venous thromboembolism (VTE) prophylaxis for patients at risk of VTE
- Chronic venous disease
- Lymphoedema

Directions of use:
- Ensure stockings are worn appropriately with the ends not rolled as this can lead to unnecessary tightness and pain
- Stockings should be worn throughout the day for the prescribed period of time, apart from when bathing or showering

DOI: 10.1201/9781003159179-17

Cautions and contraindications:
- Generally safe to use, with relatively few complications
- Poor fitting stockings may lead to discomfort and pressure sores
- Contraindications include peripheral arterial disease, localised skin infection or trauma to affected limb

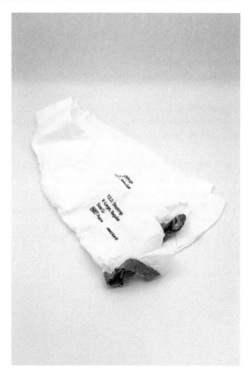

Walking aids

Description:
- Ambulatory assistive devices used to improve patient mobility and balance or to reduce weight bearing of an affected limb or limbs
- Common walking aids include canes, crutches, walkers and standing aids

Indication:
- Temporary or permanent reduction in mobility or balance of any cause
- Reduction or elimination of weight bearing following certain lower limb fractures or orthopaedic surgery

Directions of use:
- Walking aids should be prescribed and their appropriate use directed by physiotherapists or occupational therapists
- This will depend on the patients weight bearing and mobility status following through assessment

Cautions and contraindications:
- Generally safe to use, with no major contraindications
- Care must be taken as walking aids, if not used appropriately, can negatively impact on balance and lead to falls

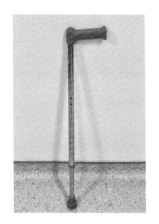

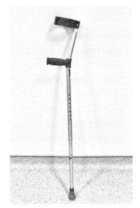

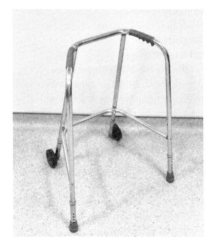

Plaster of Paris

Description:
- Moulded cast made from plaster of Paris (POP), used in the immobilisation and splinting of injured limbs including bone fractures and tendon injuries
- POP is made of calcium sulphate, which when water is added, forms a hard porous mass within 5–15 minutes, whilst producing heat
- Casts may be circumferential and placed around the whole of the affected limb, or cover only one aspect of the limb, such as a backslab

Indication:
- Conservative management of fractures of dislocations
- Soft tissue injury
- Ligament injury
- Nerve, tendon or vessel repair
- Deformity correction

Directions of use:
- Prior to casting, ensure all rings and jewellery have been removed from the distal part of the limb, and that the limb is in the optimum position for immobilisation
- Apply stockinette bandage over affected limb, ensuring whole it covers the whole length of the area to be covered by POP
- Apply one to two layers of soft padding dressing
- Measure out required length and width of POP required to immobilise the area
- Dip the POP in lukewarm water
- Place the wet POP onto the limb and gently mould to conform it to the correct position

- Hold the casted limb in the desired position until set
- Apply crepe bandage to cover POP
- Ensure comfort and adequate neurovascular status of the distal limb

Cautions and contraindications:

- Complications include deep vein thrombosis (DVT), compartment syndrome, soft tissue swelling, local pressure sores and venous congestion
- Contraindications to casting include open fractures, compartment syndrome, distal neurovascular compromise, local skin infection and severe swelling

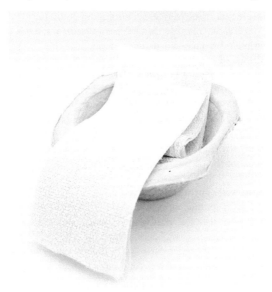

Splints

Description:

- Rigid external device applied to a limb or joint to achieve immobilisation following injury
- A variety of prefabricated splints exist to accommodate for age, size, location of affected joint and required position of immobilisation
- Splints may also be made from POP (see *Plaster of Paris*) or other thermoplastic material

Indication:

- Temporary stabilisation of fractures, ligament sprains
- Severe soft tissue injuries requiring immobilisation
- Conservative management of certain stable fractures
- Peripheral neuropathy requiring immobilisation

Directions of use:

- The injury should be appropriately assessed and the joint injury should be placed in the desired position of immobilisation
- Ensure the correct splint has been selected for the patient's age, size and joint positioning
- Apply the splint to the affected joint and secure in place ensuring stability, but avoiding excessive constriction of limb

Cautions and contraindications:

- Common complications include loss of fracture reduction, local skin irritation, post-immobilisation joint stiffness
- Rare but serious complications may include neurovascular compromise and compartment syndrome
- Thermal injury may also occur during the setting phase when using thermoplastic material such as POP or fibreglass

- Relative contraindications are include open wounds, fractures or infections and existing neurovascular compromise

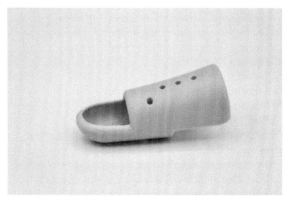

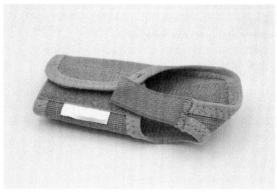

Sling

Description:
- Soft fabric immobilisation device used for the restriction of movement and provision of support and comfort in multiple upper extremity and clavicle injuries
- Various permutations of the sling exist, including the polysling, collar and cuff and broad arm sling

Indication:
- Clavicle fractures
- Acromioclavicular ligament injuries
- Shoulder dislocations
- Elbow injuries
- Forearm fractures

Directions of use:
- Instructions are described for the polysling as follows
- Place affected limb forearm into forearm support
- Secure forearm using support straps
- Pass shoulder strap around neck and adjust to required length

Cautions and contraindications:
- Complications include pressure sores following prolonged use

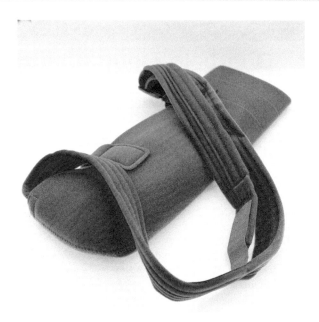

Ophthalmology

Ophthalmoscope

Description:
- Medical device used to inspect the retina and other structures of the inner eye
- Commonly comprise of a handle and a head which is equipped with an internal light source and low-power magnifying lens
- The ophthalmoscope possesses a lens wheel, filters and aperture settings, to change the diopter range, colour and shape of the light, respectively

Indication:
- Diagnosis of suspected disease affecting the fundus, e.g. hypertensive retinopathy, diabetic retinopathy, papilloedema, glaucoma and age related macular degeneration

Directions of use:
- Pupil dilation may be requires pre-procedure
- Ensure aperture set to small spot
- Focus diopter wheel until objects are in focus

DOI: 10.1201/9781003159179-18

- Check for red reflex in both eyes
- Approach patient and follow red reflex into pupil
- Examine fundus systematically in both eyes

Cautions and contraindications:

- Pupil dilation is contraindicated in patients with glaucoma as it can lead to increased intraocular pressure
- Ophthalmoscopy is a generally safe procedure

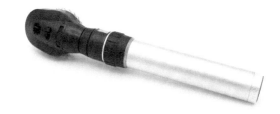

Wound care

Gauze swab

Description:
- Thin woven square piece of cotton which may be used to absorb blood or other fluids
- Gauze swabs are available in multiple sizes and may be sterile or non-sterile

Indication:
- Wound care
- Haemostasis during surgery

Directions of use:
- The uses of gauze swabs are numerous and varied
- Specific considerations regarding their use include selection of the correct size and sterility appropriate for the intended procedure

Cautions and contraindications:
- Gauze swabs are generally safe to use
- Always check for and remove any unintentionally retained swabs in the body following any invasive procedure to prevent infection risk

DOI: 10.1201/9781003159179-19

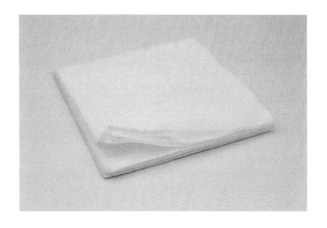

Steristrips

Description:
- Narrow adhesive strips used in the apposition of wound edges in minor wounds
- Also known as butterfly or paper stitches
- Available in multiple sizes

Indication:
- Minor injuries including lacerations and abrasions
- Postoperatively following surgical incisions

Directions of use:
- Ensure skin is cleaned and dried before application
- Select correct size steristrip and cut to appropriate size if needed
- Place steristrip overlying wound, ensuring wound edges are opposed and fully covered by the steristrip

Cautions and contraindications:
- Contraindications include large wounds where apposition cannot be achieved without sutures, profusely bleeding wounds and local skin infection

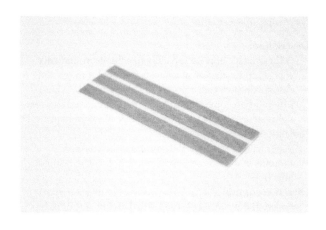

Dermal adhesive glue

Description:
- Adhesive glue applied topically to achieve wound edge apposition in small wounds with minimal skin tension
- Tissue adhesive glue consists of 2-octyl cyanoacrylate, which, when comes into contact with skin, forms a water-tight barrier that binds to the superficial epithelium

Indication:
- Superficial lacerations with minimal skin tension
- Wounds in children, to avoid need for local anaesthetic injection

Directions of use:
- Ensure the wound is cleaned, dried and haemostasis has been achieved
- Approximate the wound edges manually with slight eversion
- Apply the glue along the full length of the wound, covering both edges
- Hold the wound edges in place until the glue has dried
- For maximal strength, apply three layers of glue to the wound

Cautions and contraindications:
- Contraindications include large wounds where apposition cannot be achieved without sutures, profuse bleeding and local infection
- Upon applying the skin glue on the face, caution should be taken to avoid contact with eyes and other mucosal surfaces

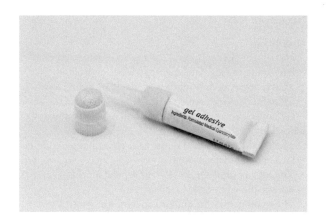

Dressings

Description:
- Material applied to wound surfaces to provide optimum environment for wound healing
- Various types of dressings are available including low adherent dressings, semipermeable films, hydrogels, alginates, foam dressings and antimicrobial dressings

Indication:
- The overarching aim of dressings is to facilitate optimum local wound management
- The type of dressing chosen will depend on the type of wound and its intended management
- The main uses of dressings include:
  - Promotion of haemostasis
  - Barrier protection from infection
  - Absorption of wound exudate
  - Provision of humidity
  - Protection from further external trauma

Directions of use:
- The most appropriate type of dressing should be chosen for the wound in question – this may require input from specialist teams such as the tissue viability nurses or the plastic surgery team
- Ensure the surrounding area is cleaned and dry
- Apply the dressing to completely cover the wound
- Dressings should be changed as scheduled, and regularly checked for signs of infection or wound breakdown

Cautions and contraindications:
- Dressings may cause allergic reactions or contact dermatitis

- Care must be taken to remove dressings in an atraumatic manner to avoid further damage to the wound and surrounding area

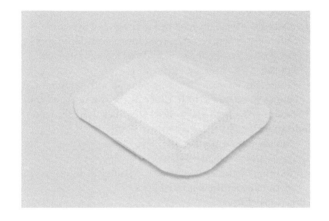

Sutures

Description:
- Sterile thread-like material used to oppose tissue in primary wound closure, provide tensile strength and promote wound healing
- A needle is typically attached to the end of the suture
- Suture types may be categorised into absorbable vs. non-absorbable, synthetic vs. natural and monofilament vs. braided
- Sutures are numbered by their diameter with thicker sutures going from 0 to 10 (10 being the thickest) and thin sutures going from 1–0 to 12–0 (12–0 being the thinnest)

Indication:
- Primary wound closure
- Bowel and vessel anastomosis
- Securing of medical equipment, e.g. surgical drains, central venous lines, arterial lines

Directions of use:
- Carefully select the appropriate suture size and type for the intended procedure
- Wear appropriate PPE when suturing
- Dispose of the needle in the sharps bin after use
- Ensure suture removal is arranged if using non-absorbable sutures

Cautions and contraindications:
- Take care when handling the needle to avoid sharps injuries
- Sutures may cause localised inflammation before they are removed

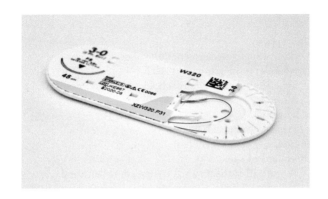

Suture kit

Description:
- Basic wound management kit to allow for suturing of wounds on the wards or in A&E
- Typically contains a needle holder, toothed forceps, suture scissors and gauze

Indication:
- Primary wound closure
- Securing drains and lines

Directions of use:
- Prepare all of the required equipment for suturing including sutures, skin preparation and dressings
- Wear appropriate PPE
- Clean wound thoroughly
- Apply evenly spaced sutures with appropriate wound apposition and minimal skin tension
- Clean and dress wound
- Give post-wound care advice including follow up for suture removal if applicable

Cautions and contraindications:
- Complications of suturing include scarring, wound infection and wound dehiscence
- Contraindications to primary wound closure include infected wounds, animal bites, significant tissue loss with skin tension on apposition

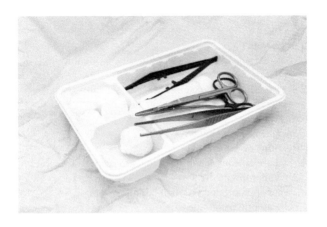

Dressing kit

Description:
- Basic wound care kit used for dressing of small wounds and minor injuries
- Typically contains gauze swabs, fold out sterile field, forceps, sterile gloves and waste bag

Indication:
- Application or change of dressing

Directions of use:
- Prepare all equipment including skin preparation solution and appropriate dressings
- Wear appropriate PPE when handling wounds
- Use aseptic technique
- Dispose of all clinical waste appropriately

Cautions and contraindications:
- Complications associated with wound care include dermatitis, infection, wound dehiscence, skin necrosis

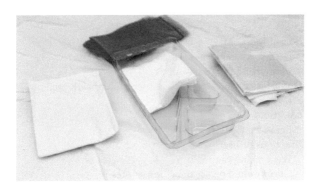

Suture removal kit

Description:
- Basic stitch removal kit used for cutting and removing suture material from wounds
- The kit typically contains a stitch cutter blade, forceps, fold out sterile field and waste bag

Indication:
- Removal of sutures

Directions of use:
- Wear appropriate PPE
- Clean wound before removing sutures
- Hold free end of suture with forceps and slide stitch cutter under suture
- Apply gentle pressure to cut suture
- Pull suture through and dispose appropriately
- Ensure all sharps are disposed of correctly following the procedure

Cautions and contraindications:
- Inappropriate use of the stitch cutter may lead to pain and bleeding around the wound site

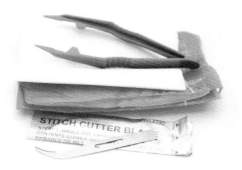

Staple remover

Description:
- Single-use device used for the atraumatic removal of surgical staples

Indication:
- Surgical staple removal

Directions of use:
- Wear appropriate PPE
- Clean wound before removing staples
- Place lower jaw under staple and squeeze handle to close the device
- This depresses the middle of the staple and removes the edges from the skin
- Ensure all sharps are disposed of correctly following the procedure

Cautions and contraindications:
- Inappropriate use of the staple remover may lead to pain and bleeding around the wound site

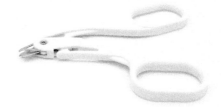

Antiseptic solution

Description:
- Chemical agents applied to the skin to disinfect the surrounding area and reduce the risk of surgical site infections
- Commonly used antiseptic agents include chlorhexidine, povidone-iodine and isopropyl alcohol

Indication:
- Cleaning of superficial wounds
- Pre-operative skin preparation
- Washout of infected wounds or abscesses

Directions of use:
- Choose most appropriate antiseptic solution for intended procedure
- Apply the solution to the area thoroughly, covering all of the surgical field or wound
- Allow the solution to dry for 2 minutes before commencing the procedure

Cautions and contraindications:
- Complications of chlorhexidine include keratitis, conjunctivitis and sensorineural deafness if in contact with the middle ear
- Povidone-iodine can stain hair and clothing, and is a known contact allergen

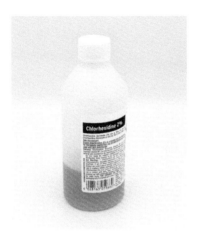

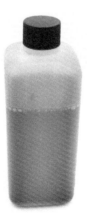

Index

Printed and bound by CPI Group (UK) Ltd, Croydon, CR0 4YY

25/10/2024

01779409-0001